I0086254

5 PILLARS TO

PEAK

PERFORMANCE

From Ordinary to Extraordinary:
The Proven Path to Winning Every Day

Joshua Euler

ISBN: 978-0-9756288-4-3

Unleash Your Potential With
The 5 Pillars To Peak Performance

You are an athlete, sportsperson, musician, dancer, performer, academic or entrepreneur, striving to be your best and setting ambitious goals. Then, one day, your Dad hands you a playbook detailing how to achieve great success.

That is how I approached this book, with my younger self in mind, wanting to give him something to help him identify where he wants to go and how to get there. So, as you read the following pages, you can expect a guide outlining the tools, strategies, and behaviours needed to be a high-performing human.

I have tried to make this more than another personal development book, instead creating an actionable guide to becoming the best version of yourself. We all deserve the opportunity to pursue our passions and live fulfilling and successful lives. If this book can help you achieve that, it will bring a great sense of purpose to my life.

Imagine a life where your brilliance shines in every endeavour, where success is not just a destination but a way of being. This book is the embodiment of that vision. It's a treasure trove of high-performance habits, mindset shifts, simplified nutritional guidance, and personal development strategies that ignite success and breed excellence.

The five pillars contain the ingredients that propel people from good to great. Each pillar is based on scientific evidence, personal and client experiences, and insights from the greats in health and high performance. I have built the five pillars into my life, and they have helped me achieve optimal health, the ability to do great things, and overcome setbacks.

I want to point out early that this isn't just about isolated areas of improvement. It's about a holistic transformation in the areas of life that will help you move the needle and power ahead. Continuous improvement is the key to long-term success.

As you journey through these pages, take your time and let each pillar sink in. Don't get to the end of the book without changing at least one habit or behaviour in your life. To help with this, at the end of each pillar, there are specific challenges to help you apply what you have learned. You don't have to try all the behaviours or strategies but pick the one/s that resonate with you and implement them into your daily routine.

Improvements come from applying what you learn, so create the changes needed to move from where you are now to where you want to be. Your current habits are perfectly designed to produce your current results. If you wish to change or improve your results, you must change your inputs (habits) to produce the desired outcomes.

The 5 Pillars To Peak Performance can be used as your compass, so keep coming back to it when things are not going according to plan and you need some guidance. It is designed to help you improve your sleep, fine-tune your training, understand nutrition, know what supplements can help your performance and well-being, overcome adversity, handle high-stress situations, create new habits and much more.

Let it guide you towards a life defined by purpose, excellence, and fulfilment. Remember, your potential knows no bounds, so let it soar.

Please now enjoy the 5 Pillars To Peak Performance.

Note To Readers: The information in this book is provided for health education purposes only. It should not be substituted for or used to alter medical therapy without your doctor's advice. For a specific health concern, consult your doctor for guidance. If you have any medical problems or injuries, consult your health professional before embarking on any dietary, supplement or exercise programs.

The author and publisher of this book disclaim any liability, loss, or risk, personal or otherwise, which is incurred as a consequence, directly or indirectly, of the use and application of any of the contents of this book. It is the reader's responsibility to ensure that any actions taken are informed by personal research and consultation with healthcare professionals.

Table of Contents

Pillar 1

Sleep And Recovery

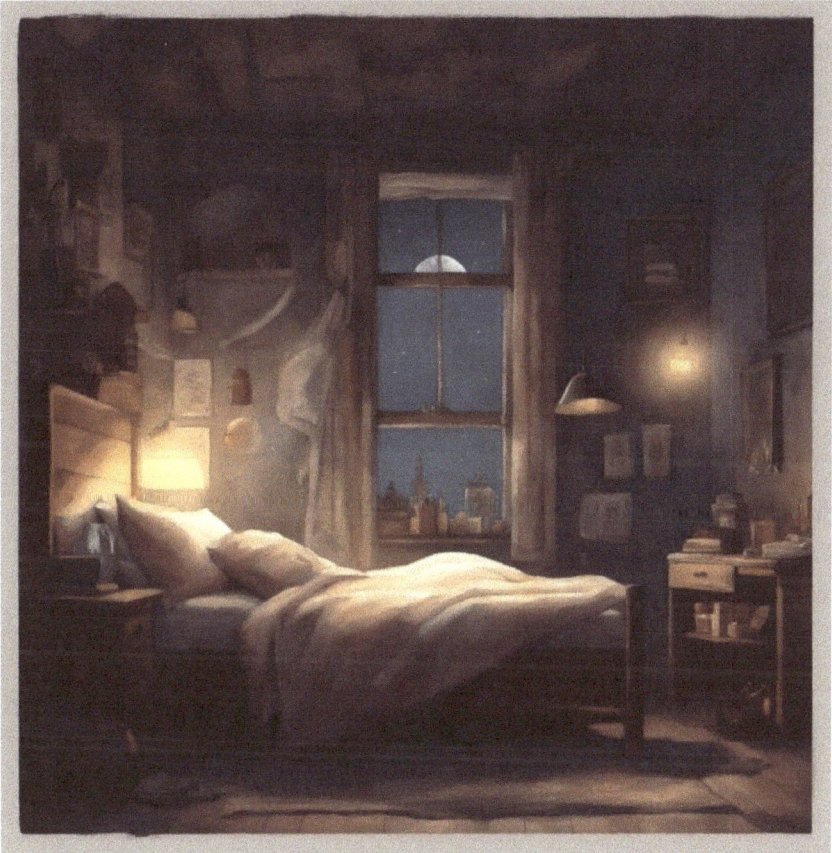

Part 1 - Sleep Is The Foundation Of Being A High Performer

I have started with sleep because all the information points to sleep as the bedrock from which a healthy body and mind are built. We have never been taught the importance of sleep and how a lack of sleep negatively impacts all performance areas. I once had the attitude, "I'll sleep when I'm dead," but that attitude was speeding up the arrival of poor health, getting injured, having an accident, and dying.

When you are young, you think you can neglect sleep and stay up late gaming, partying, or just scrolling the night away with minimal consequences the next day. This could not be further from the truth.

If you create an unhealthy sleep pattern, you will pay the price in ways you never saw coming. The negative impacts of minimal and poor-quality sleep are massive. Here is a real-world example of the benefits of extending one's sleep.

A study in Fairfax County, Virginia, USA, analysed motor vehicle accidents involving adolescents. It was conducted over two years, one year before and one year after implementing later school start times. Results show that the crash rate in 16-to-18-year-old licensed drivers decreased from 31.63 to 29.59 accidents per 1,000 drivers after the delayed start time. In contrast, the teen crash rate remained steady throughout the rest of the state.

The later start time was only 50 minutes, but it had the positive outcome of decreasing crash risks among drivers 16 to 18 years old, which has significant implications for public health and safety. Teenagers who get less sleep are more likely to make bad decisions behind the wheel, which could include distracted driving, e.g., texting, or not wearing their seatbelts. A poor night's sleep might mean the difference between safely arriving at your destination or not.

"Driving on less than 5 hours of sleep is just as dangerous as drunk driving, study finds".

We know about 20% of all vehicle crashes are caused by fatigue, so why don't we approach tired driving the same as drinking and driving?

A systematic review of 61 studies reveals very disturbing but critical information. With only 6 or 7 hours of sleep, impairment sets in, and crash likelihood surges by 30%. Pushing it further, just **one night of 4-5 hours of sleep doubles the crash risk compared to being well-rested.**

This revelation extends beyond the confines of the roads; it serves as a metaphor for the broader spectrum of our lives. A lack of sleep is deleterious to our mental and physical performance. So, it is high time we recognised that a well-rested mind and body are not optional but prerequisites for being at our best. Prioritising quality sleep is not a luxury but a foundational necessity for a high-performing life.

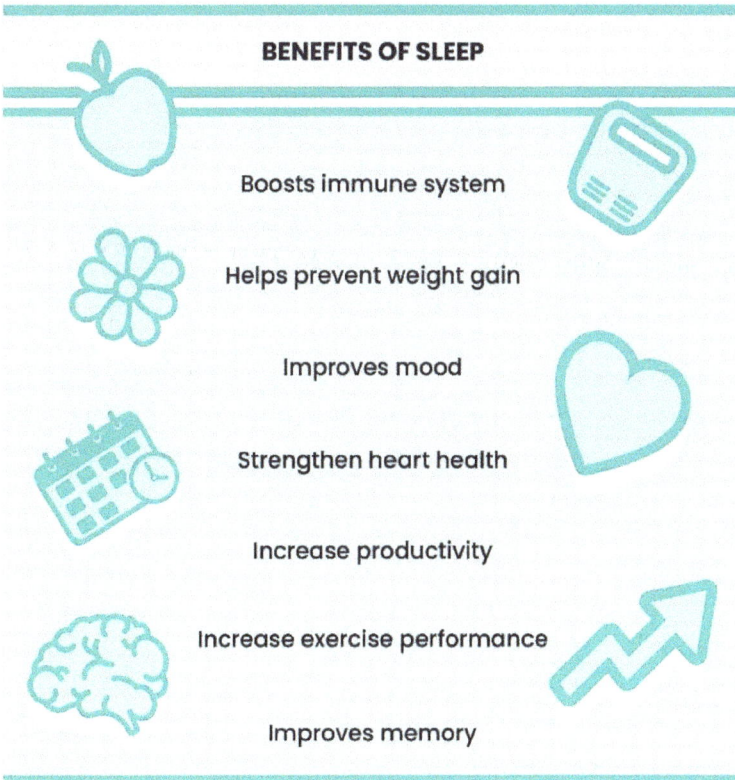

BENEFITS OF SLEEP

Boosts immune system

Helps prevent weight gain

Improves mood

Strengthen heart health

Increase productivity

Increase exercise performance

Improves memory

Positive Outcomes and Benefits Of Sleep

Reduced Risk Of Depression: Studies have found that individuals who consistently get enough sleep have a lower risk of developing depression compared to those who don't. Sleep helps regulate our mood and emotions, and chronic sleep deprivation can disrupt this regulation and lead to mood disorders.

Improved Memory and Cognitive Function: Sleep plays a crucial role in memory consolidation and cognitive function. When we sleep, our brains consolidate and store memories, which improves our ability to recall information and learn new things.

For example, a study published in the journal Sleep found that sleep extension improved cognitive performance and academic achievement in adolescents with chronic sleep reduction.

Increased Creativity: During sleep, our brains are still active and can form new connections between ideas, leading to increased creativity and problem-solving abilities.

Good-quality sleep can enhance creativity and problem-solving skills the following day, allowing you to approach challenges in new and innovative ways.

Better Stress Management: Sleep helps regulate our stress response and reduce the levels of stress hormones in our bodies. Adequate sleep can help us better manage stress and cope with demanding situations.

Better Emotional Regulation: Getting enough sleep helps us regulate our emotions and respond appropriately to situations. Sleep deprivation can lead to emotional dysregulation and cause us to overreact or respond inappropriately. Quality sleep helps regulate the parts of the brain that control our emotions, subsequently allowing us to better regulate our reactions to stressors and manage our emotions more effectively.

Enhanced Social Interactions: Getting enough good-quality sleep can help us read emotional cues and communicate effectively with others, improving our social interactions. Good-quality sleep can also improve social skills, helping people communicate effectively, regulate emotions, and build healthy relationships.

Improved Physical Health: Good-quality sleep is associated with enhanced immune function, lower inflammation levels, and a reduced risk of obesity, diabetes, and cardiovascular disease.

For example, a study published in the Paediatrics Journal found that inadequate sleep duration and poor sleep quality were associated with an increased risk of obesity in teenagers.

Improved Immune System Function: Sleep plays a vital role in the functioning of the immune system, and getting enough sleep improves the body's ability to fight off infections and diseases.

Improved Metabolism and Weight Control: Sleep regulates the hormones that control appetite and metabolism, and getting enough good-quality sleep has been linked to better weight control and a reduced risk of obesity.

Better Athletic Performance: Sleep plays a crucial role in physical recovery and muscle repair, plus getting enough good-quality sleep leads to better athletic performance and improved physical endurance.

Reduced Pain Sensitivity: Lack of sleep increases pain sensitivity, while getting enough good-quality sleep will reduce pain sensitivity.

As this extensive list illustrates, sleep is the cornerstone of high performance. Without it, our physical, emotional, and mental well-being deteriorates, limiting our ability to perform at our peak. To truly excel in both your personal and professional life, prioritising and optimising those crucial 8–9 hours of rest is non-negotiable. Sleep is not just a necessity but a superpower that fuels success.

Unveiling The Magic Of Sleep: Your Body's Superpower!

Ever wonder what happens when you drift off into dreamland? Well, it's your body's secret party time - a recovery gala, if you will! As a high performer, you're constantly learning, training, and growing, and sleep is the key to this transformative journey. Just imagine that each time you lay your head on the pillow, your body embarks on an incredible restoration, rejuvenation, and repair mission.

As diurnal creatures, humans have evolved to be most active during the day and to rest at night. This inherent pattern aligns with our circadian rhythm, the internal biological clock that governs various physiological and behavioural processes over a 24-hour cycle.

Maintaining a regular sleep-wake cycle is crucial for synchronising this rhythm and promoting overall health and well-being. Exposure to sunlight early in the morning plays a pivotal role in this process, as it signals to the brain that it's time to wake up and initiates a cascade of hormonal and neurotransmitter changes that promote alertness and activity during the day.

This exposure to natural light helps regulate the timing of sleep and wakefulness, ensuring a robust and well-aligned circadian rhythm. Therefore, establishing a consistent routine of waking up at the same time each day and getting sunlight in the morning is a cornerstone for supporting a healthy sleep-wake cycle and optimising overall performance throughout the day.

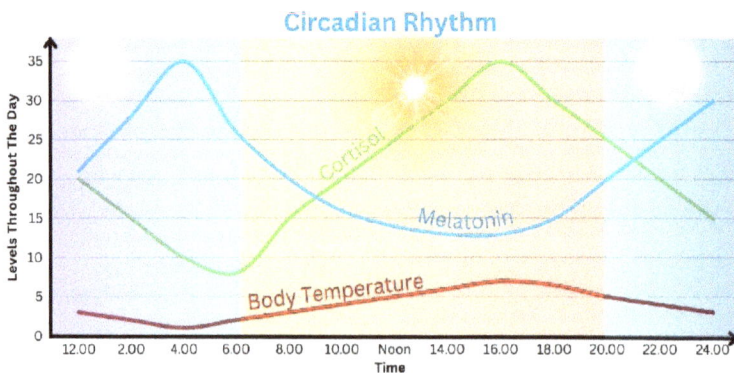

Circadian Rhythm

What Really Goes On When We Sleep

Let's explore the amazing processes that your body and brain perform each night. Normal human sleep comprises two main types: non-rapid eye movement (non-REM) and rapid eye movement (REM) sleep.

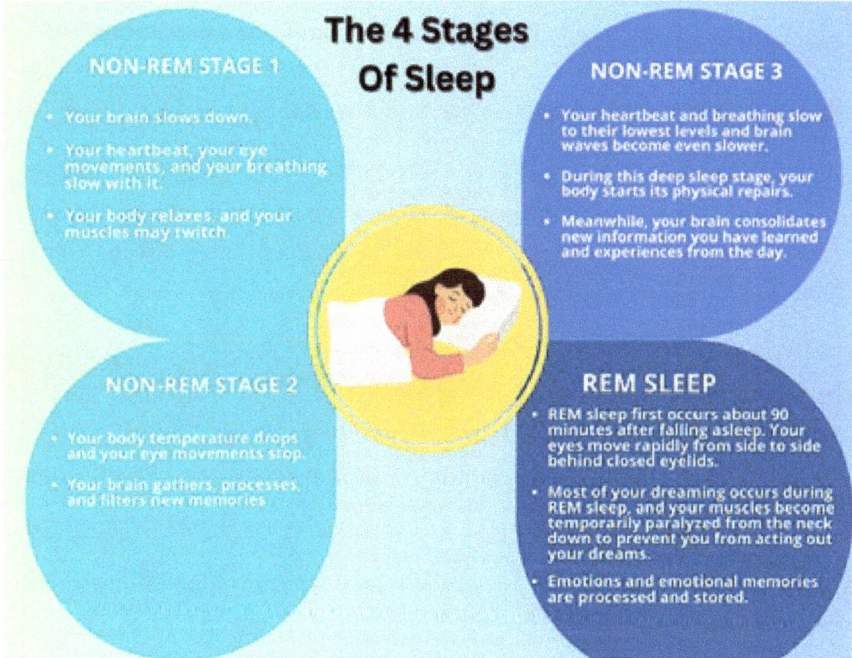

The 4 Stages Of Sleep

NON-REM STAGE 1

- Your brain slows down.
- Your heartbeat, your eye movements, and your breathing slow with it.
- Your body relaxes, and your muscles may twitch.

NON-REM STAGE 3

- Your heartbeat and breathing slow to their lowest levels and brain waves become even slower.
- During this deep sleep stage, your body starts its physical repairs.
- Meanwhile, your brain consolidates new information you have learned and experiences from the day.

NON-REM STAGE 2

- Your body temperature drops and your eye movements stop.
- Your brain gathers, processes, and filters new memories

REM SLEEP

- REM sleep first occurs about 90 minutes after falling asleep. Your eyes move rapidly from side to side behind closed eyelids.
- Most of your dreaming occurs during REM sleep, and your muscles become temporarily paralyzed from the neck down to prevent you from acting out your dreams.
- Emotions and emotional memories are processed and stored.

Non-REM sleep is divided into three stages, representing a continuum from 'light' sleep in stages 1 and 2 to 'deep' sleep in stage 3. Non-REM sleep is fundamental for cognitive functions such as learning, distillation of new information, and physical repair. Each cycle of non-REM sleep paves the way for the subsequent REM phase, with these cycles repeating throughout the night.

During REM sleep, the brain becomes highly active, almost mirroring its state during wakefulness, which is why we have vivid dreams. REM is characterised by rapid eye movements, increased respiration rate, and temporary paralysis of the muscles from the neck down, which prevents us from acting out our dreams.

REM sleep is critical in emotional regulation, memory consolidation, and problem-solving. It's a period of intense brain activity during which the brain processes and integrates experiences from the day into long-term memory. It's a period of neural pathways strengthening, supporting learning and memory.

The cyclical alternation between REM and non-REM sleep throughout the night underscores sleep's intricate architecture and highlights its profound impact on our cognitive, emotional, and physical well-being.

As you can see, each stage is responsible for conducting essential functions. This means that if you get to bed late and/or need to get up early and subsequently miss stages of your night's sleep, there will be varying consequences the next day.

This is why it is so important to establish a regular sleep routine as a high performer. It only takes a few days with less than 7 hours of sleep, and you will start to see impaired cognition, poor learning and memory consolidation, emotional control, and not recovering well from training sessions.

Sleep is far from a passive state; it's an incredibly dynamic and vital process where your body and mind perform critical functions that keep you healthy, balanced, and ready to tackle the day ahead. From repairing tissues to processing emotions, sleep is your body's version of a 24/7 operating system that shifts into high gear when you rest. Let's dive into the essential tasks your body undertakes while you sleep and why optimising this nightly reset is key to your overall well-being.

Cellular Repair: The Night-Time Construction Crew

Do you know how a city's maintenance crew often works at night to avoid disrupting the day's hustle and bustle? Similarly, your body does the same. It releases higher growth hormone levels during sleep, a critical ingredient in repairing muscles and bones. It's like a construction crew working diligently under the moonlight to ensure the roads (your body) are ready for the next day!

Memory Consolidation: The Brain's Night Shift

While dreaming, your brain is busy sorting, filing, and processing your day's experiences. While you sleep, your brain downloads the information you have learned and creates new neural connections to strengthen your memories. Consider it like your brain's administrative assistant, meticulously organising your day's learning and lessons.

Hormone Regulation: The Chemist

Sleep plays a crucial role in regulating various hormones in the body. This intricate hormonal dance during sleep is essential for maintaining overall health and well-being. Disruptions in sleep patterns or insufficient sleep can lead to hormonal imbalances, affecting mood, cognitive function, immune response, libido and metabolic health.

Detoxication: The Brain's Cleaning Service

Just as you need to clean your room, your brain must clear the clutter and keep the space clean. Sleep calls in your brain's cleaning service, removing toxins and waste accumulated throughout the day to keep everything running smoothly.

Immune System Support: Your Body's Personal Army

During sleep, your immune system transforms into a defence fortress, producing cytokines, proteins that help fight infections and inflammation. It's your body's army, preparing for battle while you're sleeping peacefully.

Emotional Regulation: The Therapist

During REM sleep, the brain becomes highly active, triggering a fascinating process akin to a therapy session. It's as if the mind is a therapist, helping you understand the emotional weight of different events. During this stage, the brain might replay scenarios, providing an opportunity to process and understand emotions, contributing to emotional resilience and well-being.

Without REM Sleep, there is no emotional processing, which is a significant factor in most mental health conditions. This relationship between insufficient sleep and poor mental health should motivate anyone to focus on optimising their sleep.

The Impact Of Sleep Interventions On Athletic Performance

Many studies have examined various aspects of sleep and athletic performance. Analysing the most relevant twenty-five studies encompassing many sports and interventions, the data pinpoints that extending sleep, sleep banking or introducing napping is very effective for enhancing cognitive and physical performance.

Getting 7-8 hours of quality sleep positively affects athletic performance, but a lack of sleep is more detrimental. Mediocre performance ensues when athletes do not get adequate sleep. Below are examples of what happens to athletic performance when the subject does not get sufficient quality sleep.

Decreased Accuracy - After sleep deprivation, male and female tennis players decreased serve accuracy by up to 53% compared to performance after normal sleep.

Quicker Exhaustion - In a study of male runners and volleyball players, both groups could not maintain performance levels and fatigued faster after sleep deprivation.

Decreased Reaction Time - A lack of sleep adversely affected reaction time in a studied group of male collegiate athletes.

Slower Decision-Making - A lack of sleep impacts executive functions. Choices such as passing or kicking the ball or deciding on the best shot to hit can be more difficult or made too late.

Risk of Injury - Research on middle and high school athletes revealed that a chronic lack of sleep is associated with increased rates of injury.

Risk of Illness - Poor sleep habits are associated with lower resistance to illness, such as the common cold, which results in missed training sessions and game time.

Approach Your Endeavours Like An Athlete

No matter your field - be it music, performing arts, entrepreneurship, medicine, or coding - success demands the same disciplined approach a high-performing athlete takes. Why? Because performing at your best isn't just about talent; it's about consistency, resilience, and intentional habits.

Athletes understand that sleep, recovery, nutrition, and exercise aren't optional; they're non-negotiable pillars of their success. The same applies to you. If you want to perform at your best, you must prioritise these foundational elements to optimise your physical and mental capabilities.

Consider this: Your current habits are perfectly designed to produce your current results. Hence, if your results aren't where you want them to be, it's time to reevaluate your inputs. Change your habits, and you'll change your outcomes. Adopt an athlete's approach, and you'll be equipped to reach new levels of success in whatever you pursue.

How To Make Sure You Can Perform At Your Best.

Increase Sleep Duration: Studies implementing sleep extension consistently demonstrated enhanced performance outcomes, suggesting that extending sleep duration by 46–113 minutes for more than three nights is the recommendation for athletes habitually sleeping around 7 hours. Athletes reported needing around 8.3 hours of sleep but often fell short, emphasising the importance of extending sleep duration to bridge this gap and improve their performance.

Napping: General performance outcomes decline when sleep is restricted to less than five hours. However, studies have shown that napping can effectively restore performance to baseline levels. Following a night of partial sleep restriction, research indicated that even a 20-minute nap effectively restored performance to levels comparable to a night of normal sleep. 90-minute naps showed better improvements, but if you have 30 minutes to lay down and close your eyes, it can be a game changer.

Sleep Banking: This is the practice of intentionally increasing sleep duration before anticipated sleep disruptions and is a valuable tool for athletes facing travel, time zone changes, or unfamiliar environments. Research shows that extending sleep by 1–2 hours per night in the days leading up to an event can mitigate the negative effects of sleep deprivation, preserving both cognitive and physical performance. To maximise the benefits, ensure the additional sleep is of high quality by maintaining a consistent sleep routine and environment. Sleep banking serves as a proactive strategy to sustain peak performance during demanding schedules.

Sleep Behaviours: Sleep hygiene (practices and habits that promote healthy and restful sleep) interventions such as removing electronic devices from the bedroom demonstrated no significant impact on recovery or cognitive performance. However, optimising the sleep environment, e.g., temperature and darkness, combined with mindfulness practices improves sleep outcomes.

Using a sauna or spa before bed can enhance sleep duration and quality. A recent study found that frequent sauna use was associated with better sleep quality, including longer sleep duration and better sleep quality. Similarly, a spa or a hot bath before bedtime has also led to improved sleep. Heat-induced relaxation and the subsequent decrease in core body temperature after getting out of the heat help facilitate sleep onset and promote more restful sleep.

What To Do If You Cannot Sleep?

You should not stay in bed for long if you are awake and going stir-crazy. Our brain is a remarkably effective prediction and association device. Hence, the brain will learn behaviour patterns and compute that the bedroom is about being awake. So, getting up and moving to another room is worth trying. The room must be dimly lit, so do not turn on all the lights. Just read or listen to a book (preferably a boring one) or melodic music - no screens, no phones!

Only when you're sleepy do you go back to bed. That way, your brain relearns to associate your bedroom with sleep rather than wakefulness.

Another thing you can do if you don't want to get up and go to a different room is follow a guided sleep-focused meditation. This will allow you to get out of your head and stop focusing on those worrying thoughts.

You can also try sleep-inducing white noise, such as rainforest sounds or bubbling streams. Many options are available, so if one does not work, try something else and never give up on getting a good night's sleep.

Another effective method is to create an adventure or fairytale to let your mind wander and escape the situation or person stealing your sleep. Creating this narrative turns off the analytical, self-critical part of the brain and engages the creative, non-judgemental centre. This allows you to disentangle yourself from the recurring thoughts keeping you awake.

The underlying principle is to redirect your focus away from the emotionally charged thoughts keeping you awake. When replaying the same scenario repeatedly, redirecting and stopping can be challenging. Engaging in non-critical creative thinking may effectively redirect attention, calming the mind and facilitating falling asleep. So don't just lie awake, looking at the clock, stressing that you must get up in 3 hours. Put any or all of these strategies to work and do whatever you can to get back those potentially lost hours of sleep.

If you've established a sleep-friendly pre-bed routine and still struggle to get quality sleep, it may be time to think outside the box. Innovative therapies such as Sleep Restriction Therapy, Cognitive Behavioural Therapy for Insomnia (CBT-I), and Light Therapy have shown promising results in improving sleep patterns. These methods work by adjusting the body's internal clock, optimising sleep efficiency, and reinforcing natural circadian rhythms.

For individuals with sleep apnea (when you stop breathing while asleep due to no airflow), certain adjustments can make a significant difference. Many find it difficult to sleep on their back due to how this position affects the airways. When lying on your back, gravity pulls the tongue and soft tissues downward, often leading to partial or complete airway obstruction. This blockage disrupts breathing, causing frequent awakenings and lowering oxygen levels throughout the night.

Switching to side-sleeping can help alleviate these obstructions, as it allows gravity to move the tongue and soft tissues away from the throat rather than into it. Some individuals also benefit from using a specially designed mouthguard that gently brings the lower jaw forward, which helps keep the airway open and minimises blockages. For many, combining side-sleeping with this supportive mouthguard can help create a more consistent and restful sleep.

Excess weight, particularly around the neck and chest, can exacerbate sleep apnea by increasing pressure on the airways. In people with obesity, fat deposits in the upper respiratory tract narrow the airway, and decreased muscle activity in this region increases the likelihood of airway collapse during sleep. The constant wakings this causes trap individuals in a cycle of fragmented, shallow sleep that prevents deep, restorative rest.

Moreover, the cycle of poor sleep and weight gain can reinforce itself. Broken sleep disrupts hormonal balance, particularly the hormones leptin and ghrelin, which regulate hunger and satiety. As sleep quality declines, leptin levels drop (reducing the sense of fullness), and ghrelin levels rise (increasing hunger), often intensifying cravings for high-carb, high-calorie foods. This hormonal imbalance can make it harder to manage weight, creating a vicious cycle that exacerbates sleep apnea symptoms.

Even modest weight loss can help alleviate pressure on the airway, improve breathing, and enhance overall sleep quality. For those with sleep apnea, combining weight management with side sleeping and a specialised mouthguard that supports the jaw can be a powerful strategy to break this cycle and allow deeper, more restorative sleep.

If you are struggling with your health due to poor sleep, don't hesitate to seek help from a health professional who understands the importance of sleep and can help implement these therapies.

As we conclude this exploration of all the fantastic things sleep helps us accomplish, a pivotal question arises: Can you offset a sleep debt by sleeping longer on another day?

It's an enticing notion to think you can repay a sleep debt by indulging in extra slumber on the weekend, attempting to catch up on the lack of sleep lost during the week. However, the reality is starkly different. Sleep doesn't work like a bank, where you can accumulate a debt and pay it off later.

Consider this - If you were deprived of an entire night's sleep, stripped of a full eight hours and provided ample time the following night, you might sleep longer, yet the stark truth is that you won't reclaim all that you've lost. No matter how much sleep you indulge in during the subsequent night, the brain lacks the mechanism to recover the sleep debt that has been accrued fully. Restoring those lost hours and benefits that come with them is beyond the brain's capacity.

This concept is foundational in understanding the complexities of sleep. It's not merely about clocking in hours but also about maintaining a consistent and healthy sleep pattern to ensure the brain and body function optimally.

Consider sleeping your secret weapon. It manages the night work crew, which helps rebuild muscle and clears away the waste built up during the day. It is the mastermind behind your memory and the guardian of your emotional health.

After a long day, there is nothing quite like the restful embrace of sleep. Let's now look at the best ways to start and finish your day to ensure you can achieve the perfect night's sleep.

Part 2 - Transform Your Sleep - Start And Finish Your Day Right!

Sleep can be that elusive creature that can evade us when we need it most. But when you get it, it is your secret weapon. It's the cloak of invincibility you wear to face the world.

How do you capture this mythical beast? Well, it's all in the routine and hard work done during the day. Here is your guide to getting to the land of sweet dreams and bright mornings.

High Performers Morning Routine

Get Direct Sunlight: Sunlight is your body's natural alarm clock and aligns with our natural circadian rhythm. So, getting direct natural light into your eyes within the first 30 minutes of waking up sets your body's internal clock ticking. Seeing sunlight starts your diurnal clock, so 16 hours later, when it's time to go to bed, you feel sleepy and ready to hit the hay.

When natural sunlight isn't available, such as on overcast days or during early mornings in winter, using a light therapy box can be an effective alternative. These devices are designed to mimic the brightness of sunlight, typically providing a light intensity of around 10,000 lux, which is similar to outdoor light on a clear day.

Hydrate: A glass of water helps rehydrate and stimulates saliva production, which is essential for maintaining oral health. Drinking water also helps move bacteria from your mouth into the gastrointestinal (GI) tract. The stomach's acidic environment can neutralise many harmful bacteria and improve the diversity of bacteria in your gut microbiome.

Delay Your Morning Coffee: While coffee is a cherished morning ritual for many, drinking it immediately upon waking can disrupt your body's natural rhythm, particularly the processes involving cortisol and adenosine. Delaying your first cup of coffee can optimise your energy throughout the day and avoid unwanted crashes.

I know this will be a hard sell for many people, so let me explain why.

Adenosine and Sleep Pressure: Adenosine is a neurotransmitter that builds up throughout the day as a by-product of energy use, creating "sleep pressure" that signals your body it's time to rest. Overnight, adenosine levels naturally drop as they are cleared away. Upon waking, your body experiences a natural rise in cortisol, a hormone that promotes alertness and mood. This cortisol spike not only wakes you up but also aids in clearing residual adenosine, helping you feel refreshed and alert at the start of the day.

Caffeine's Mechanism: Caffeine is an adenosine receptor antagonist, meaning it binds to adenosine receptors in the brain without activating them, temporarily blocking the drowsiness adenosine induces. However, caffeine doesn't reduce adenosine, it simply masks its effects. As caffeine wears off, residual adenosine can quickly rebind to receptors, which may lead to a rebound sleepiness effect.

Impact of Caffeine on the Natural Cortisol Spike: The body's natural cortisol spike, occurring within 30-45 minutes of waking, serves as an internal wake-up signal to help clear adenosine. Drinking coffee immediately after waking interferes with this natural cortisol peak, replacing your body's built-in wakefulness mechanisms with an artificial stimulant. Since caffeine doesn't clear adenosine, the leftover adenosine remains in your system and can quickly rebind to receptors as caffeine levels drop, often resulting in feeling fatigued shortly after.

Avoiding the Afternoon Crash: Delaying caffeine intake until after the natural cortisol peak enables your body to complete its morning alertness cycle without interference. This approach helps maintain stable energy levels, reducing the need for additional caffeine later in the day, which, if consumed too late, can disrupt sleep and lead to a cycle of poor rest and caffeine dependence.

Waiting 60-90 minutes after waking before consuming caffeine allows cortisol to peak naturally and support adenosine clearance. This minimises the risk of energy dips and helps maintain consistent energy throughout the day.

Move Your Body: Exercising in the morning is like jumpstarting your body and mind. It gets your blood flowing, releases endorphins, and boosts energy naturally, leaving you more alert and ready to take on the day. Morning workouts also set a positive tone, increasing the likelihood of making healthier choices throughout the day, such as better nutrition and improved focus.

Another key benefit is consistency. Morning exercise reduces the risk of skipping your workout due to unexpected distractions or responsibilities later in the day. Fewer interruptions make it easier to establish a regular routine. Exercising in the morning outdoors provides additional perks. Sunlight exposure early in the day helps regulate your circadian rhythm, improving sleep quality and aiding Vitamin D synthesis.

Engaging in steady-state cardio in the morning, especially in a fasted state, can enhance fat mobilisation and oxidation. With lower glycogen stores, your body is more likely to utilise stored fat for energy. Additionally, light activities like jogging or walking can improve insulin sensitivity, aiding in better blood sugar control.

For those who prefer training later in the day, incorporating even a short morning walk can offer similar benefits, boosting mood and providing a dose of fresh air and natural light.

Practice Gratitude, Meditation, or Breathing Exercises: If you are not exercising in the morning, I strongly recommend starting your day with a self-priming activity. Pick the activity that creates a clear mind and direction for your day. Write down things you're grateful for, meditate, do breath work or even set your intentions for the day. It's like a warm-up for your mind before it faces the day. Spend 15-30 minutes setting yourself up to have a great day.

Avoid Checking Your Phone: Hold off diving into the digital world. Don't deplete your dopamine stores before walking out the door. Take time to do the above activities before getting caught up in the grip of social media, TV and news.

Evening Routine - How To Prepare For A Wonderful Night's Sleep.

Avoid Bright Light Before Bedtime: Engaging with bright screens, whether scrolling through your phone, gaming or working on a computer, directly disrupts your body's ability to prepare for sleep. These devices emit blue light, which suppresses the production of melatonin, the hormone that signals to your brain that it's time to sleep. Research shows that blue light has the most potent effect on delaying melatonin release, making it harder to fall asleep and reducing the overall quality of your sleep.

To safeguard your sleep:

- Minimize screen use at least 60–90 minutes before bed.

- Use blue light filters or night mode on electronic devices if you must use them in the evening.

- Opt for warmer, dimmer lighting, such as bedside lamps or candles, to create a relaxing environment.

These small adjustments protect melatonin production and help your body and mind transition naturally into a state of rest, setting the stage for deep and restorative sleep.

Avoid Caffeine and Alcohol Before Bedtime: These substances are like unwanted guests at your sleep party. While caffeine is a well-known stimulant that can keep you awake, alcohol can also disrupt your sleep cycle. Although alcohol might initially make you feel drowsy, it interferes with REM sleep, the most restorative stage, and leads to fragmented sleep and frequent awakenings. This disruption can leave you feeling groggy and tired the next day, undermining the quality of your rest and overall well-being. To ensure a more restful and rejuvenating sleep, it's best to avoid caffeine and alcohol in the hours leading up to bedtime.

Create a Relaxing Bedtime Routine: Don't miss your time to unwind. Set a bedtime reminder if you are bad at switching off. Put a timer on your wall to cut power to your TV or WIFI, and start winding down at least 30 minutes before trying to sleep. Take a warm shower or bath, listen to calming music or read a book. Set yourself up for a great night's sleep.

Keep Your Bedroom Cool, Dark, and Quiet: Your sleep environment plays a crucial role in achieving high-quality sleep. A cool room is essential for quality sleep because your core body temperature needs to drop by 1–2°C to initiate and maintain deep, restorative sleep. This natural cooling process helps your body transition into the deeper stages of sleep, where critical functions like cellular repair, memory consolidation, and hormonal regulation occur.

Keeping your room cool, ideally between 16 and 20 degrees Celsius (65 degrees Fahrenheit), supports this temperature drop, making it easier to fall asleep and stay asleep. A cool environment also prevents overheating, which can disrupt your sleep cycles and reduce overall sleep quality.

This is where using thermal relaxation techniques, like using a sauna or hot bath 30 – 60 minutes before bed, can further enhance this effect. These activities temporarily raise your body temperature, and as your body cools down afterwards, it triggers the natural drop in core temperature needed for sleep onset.

Additionally, ensure your room is completely dark and free from distracting light sources, even from small LEDs. Cover these lights and aim for total darkness, so dark that you can't see your hand in front of your face. Combine this with a quiet environment to create the ultimate sleep sanctuary for deep, restorative sleep.

So there you have it - the dos and don'ts for capturing the best night's sleep. Try these tactics, and before you know it, you'll be a high-performing sleep machine.

Sleep Tools To Promote And Support Quality Sleep

If you are doing all of these behaviours to improve your sleep and are still not getting 7-9 hours of deep, restful sleep, here are some ideas, tools and supplements that help you fall asleep and improve the quality and duration of your sleep.

Sleep Equipment.

I will start with the most overlooked and underappreciated method of improving sleep: ensuring you have a good-quality mattress and pillow. We spend eight hours per night on our mattresses, so don't neglect it.

A good mattress lasts, on average, 8-10 years; however, pay attention to your body's cues. If it is too hard or soft and you can't get comfortable, waking up with aches and pains, you may need to replace your mattress sooner. If you've recently slept somewhere else, like a friend's house or hotel, and you feel more comfortable than in your bed at home, these are all signs your mattress isn't what it needs to be. A worn-out mattress can significantly impact your sleep quality and overall health.

A good pillow is equally important as it supports your head and neck, maintaining proper alignment with the spine, which helps prevent neck pain and reduces tossing and turning. Your neck has a natural forward curve that helps support your head's weight when standing or sitting. Maintaining this position is essential when sleeping. Adjustable pillows for your bed could help your neck stay in place. They prevent excess movement and an uncomfortable posture. Placing a pillow between your legs or under your knees could also help with spinal alignment. It may take the pressure off your hips and lower back, increasing comfort.

Different pillows, such as memory foam, latex, and even buckwheat, cater to various sleeping positions and personal preferences. I started using a latex pillow a few years ago, and I'm now onto my second, as they are soft yet supportive. It is also worth replacing your pillow every one to two years.

The next is high-quality sheets that help regulate body temperature by allowing air to circulate, preventing heat and moisture build-up that can disrupt sleep. Great options, like cotton or bamboo, feel great and are not too expensive.

Lastly, a small but worthwhile adjustment is to avoid tucking in the bottom of your sheets too tightly, especially on the side. Allowing your feet to move freely can enhance comfort and circulation, preventing feelings of restriction that might disrupt sleep. This adjustment can make a significant difference in overall comfort and sleep quality.

Supplements

Apigenin (Chamomile tea): The compound in chamomile tea is believed to assist with sleep. Apigenin is a flavonoid that is found in various plants, including chamomile. It has been shown to have sedative effects and can bind to specific receptors in the brain that promote relaxation and sleep.

Valerian root: This herbal supplement has been used for centuries as a natural sleep aid. It has been shown to improve sleep quality and reduce the time it takes to fall asleep.

L-theanine: An amino acid found in green tea that has a calming effect on the body. Supplementing with L-theanine has been shown to improve sleep quality and reduce the time it takes to fall asleep, particularly in individuals with anxiety.

Ashwagandha: Ashwagandha has been used for over 3,000 years to relieve stress, increase energy levels, and improve concentration. More recently, it has been found to enhance overall sleep quality, making it easier for individuals to fall asleep and stay asleep longer, possibly due to its effects on stress reduction.

Passionflower: A plant traditionally used for its calming and sleep-inducing properties. It's often recommended as a natural remedy for anxiety, insomnia, and related sleep disorders. The proposed mechanisms behind its effects include increased levels of gamma-aminobutyric acid (GABA) in the brain. This neurotransmitter helps regulate mood and can decrease neuronal activity, leading to relaxation and better sleep.

Glycine: An amino acid, glycine has the potential to improve sleep quality by affecting body temperature regulation and calming the nervous system. Some studies suggest it can help individuals fall asleep faster.

Magnesium: Magnesium is the hidden gem that plays a big role in calming your nervous system and promoting relaxation through enhanced

GABA activity. This mineral also eases muscle tension and promotes physical relaxation. Magnesium works harmoniously with melatonin to ensure a seamless sleep-wake cycle and help you achieve a blissful night's rest. You will find a list of the different forms of magnesium and their benefits in the nutrition section.

Sleep Apps

Selecting a sleep app that aligns with your needs is crucial for improving sleep quality. Sleep apps offer diverse functionalities catering to various aspects of sleep. While some apps focus on monitoring sleep patterns and cycles, others prioritise relaxation techniques or provide access to expert advice.

To make an informed choice, consider what aspects of sleep you want to prioritise and explore how these app features can support your unique sleep goals. Here are **five top-rated apps** to get you started.

Headspace: Known for meditation and mindfulness exercises, Headspace includes sleep-specific meditations, breathing exercises, and wind-down routines to help relax the mind and body before sleep.

Calm: This app offers sleep stories, soothing music, guided meditations, and soundscapes to promote relaxation and better sleep. Calm's Sleep Stories are narrated by well-known voices to aid in sleep preparation.

Sleep Cycle: Utilising your phone's accelerometer, Sleep Cycle tracks sleep patterns and wakes you during your lightest sleep phase, aiming to prevent grogginess. It also provides a detailed sleep analysis.

BetterSleep: Discover your chronotype, track your sleep and create effective bedtime routines that draw from our rich audio collection, guided stories, and relaxation practices.

ShutEye: This app analyses the sounds and movements recorded by your phone's microphone and produces sleep status information using artificial intelligence algorithms. At the same time, selected sleep recordings, such as snoring, are available for your listening and sharing.

Journaling

Doing this before bed can be an effective pre-sleep routine to improve sleep quality. The practice involves writing down thoughts, emotions, or events from the day, providing an opportunity to process and release stress or worries before bedtime.

Research in psychology supports the idea that expressive writing, including journaling, can have psychological and emotional benefits. Studies have shown that expressive writing might reduce intrusive and avoidant thoughts, potentially improving sleep.

Here's how journaling can aid in a more restful night's sleep.

Stress Reduction: Journaling is a mental unloading process, allowing individuals to empty their minds of racing thoughts, concerns, or anxieties. This can help reduce stress and anxiety, enabling a more relaxed state before sleep.

Enhanced Problem Solving: Writing about daily challenges or concerns can often lead to a clearer perspective or potential solutions, reducing the mind's tendency to ruminate on unresolved issues while trying to sleep.

Gratitude Practice: Focusing on positive experiences from the day or things to be grateful for can foster a more positive mindset and promote feelings of contentment and relaxation before sleep.

Emotional Freedom Tapping (EFT)

Commonly known as tapping, this technique combines acupressure and psychological principles to alleviate stress and anxiety, which are common obstacles to restful sleep. By gently tapping on specific meridian points on the face and body, combined with focusing on negative emotions or physical discomfort, tapping helps to release energy blockages and promote relaxation.

To use tapping to help you sleep, you need to tap, identify the stress or anxiety you're experiencing, rate its intensity, and create a set-up statement. For example, "Even though I have this problem (while at the same time affirming self-acceptance), I deeply and completely accept myself." Here is an overview of the EFT Process.

State how you feel (be honest) and pair this with a self-acceptance statement. For example, "Even though I'm really anxious about work tomorrow, I accept I feel this way." State this while tapping on the side of your hand. Rate the discomfort on a scale from 0 to 10 (0 = no distress, 10 = complete distress).

Now, work through the 8 EFT points while saying the phrase. After tapping all 8 spots, take a breath and re-rate your distress out of 10. Continue this cycle until your distress levels are down towards 0. Now, transition to a new positive outcome statement to help fall asleep, e.g., I trust my body to get deep and restorative sleep.

Tapping takes some practice so try it out during the day when you're not under pressure to fall asleep. This allows you to become familiar with the process and more comfortable using it at night when you need it most.

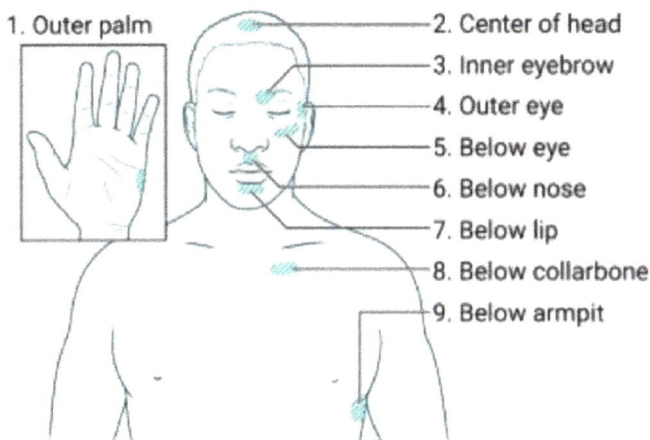

1. Outer palm
2. Center of head
3. Inner eyebrow
4. Outer eye
5. Below eye
6. Below nose
7. Below lip
8. Below collarbone
9. Below armpit

How to Make Sleep Your Superpower!

Start by setting a sleep schedule, and if you are a coffee lover, put as much importance on it as the morning coffee, and you will never miss it. Aim for the same bedtime as often as possible. Next, design a bedtime routine that's as relaxing as a spa treatment. Think of warm baths, calming music, or an enjoyable book. Then, create the perfect sleep environment that is as inviting as a luxury resort, with comfortable pillows, cosy blankets, and a quiet, dark room. Finally, write down your thoughts or express gratitude for the things you have in your life and then open your preferred sleep app. Play your sleep-inducing music or sounds, and let the app track your night's sleep as you fall asleep.

When you wake up, assess how you feel and compare it to the data on your app so you can review what happened throughout the night and continue to improve your bedtime routine and environment. Just be aware that sometimes you might not get a good sleep score but feel well-rested. Don't let your sleep score affect how you think and approach your day. Use it as a tool; don't let it dictate how you approach your day.

But here's the tricky part - avoiding things that keep you glued to that screen and your brain on high alert. Just because you have your phone by your bed, do not allow yourself to mindlessly scroll on your favourite platform when the lights should be off. Highly stimulating screen time before trying to sleep is like a flashing billboard disturbing your peaceful drive to slumberland. This short-term pleasure-seeking is robbing your long-term success, so turn off the electronic device and get a good night's rest.

"Sleep is the magic that transforms effort into excellence. It restores your body, sharpens your mind, and fuels your ambition, laying the foundation upon which your best self is built. Without it, even your greatest efforts will fall short of their true potential."

Part 3 - Unlocking Peak Performance With The Right Recovery Strategies

In the world of high performance, optimising recovery becomes a non-negotiable aspect of the training regimen. If you are pushing hard across multiple areas of life, engaging in some form of recovery will allow you to keep that level of performance up.

It is important to recognise that most improvements happen after the workout, training, practice, or study session. This is why sleep is your number one recovery tool, followed by nutrition and hydration. However, there are a variety of recovery tools that can be used to improve recovery and performance. These recovery strategies vary in effectiveness, as seen in the recovery pyramid below.

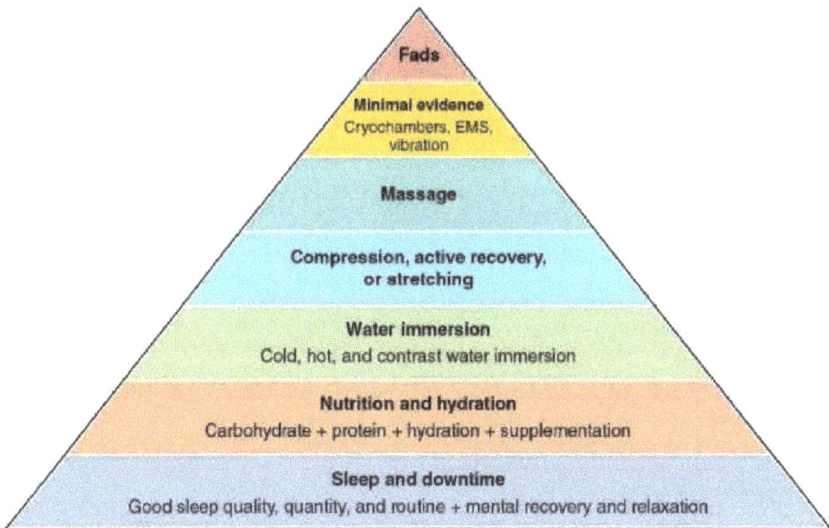

Image from NSCA's Essentials of Sport Science

We have discussed the importance of sleep and will cover nutrition, hydration, and supplementation in the following pillars. So, let's discuss the other reliable recovery tools: water immersion, compression, active recovery, stretching and massage.

Water Immersion

This popular recovery method includes cold-water immersion, hot-water immersion, and contrast (hot-cold) therapy.

Cold Water Immersion involves submerging your body (excluding the head) in cold water, typically between 5°C and 15°C, for up to 20 minutes.

Why do it? Cold Water Immersion works by constricting blood vessels, which helps push out metabolic waste products and reduce swelling and inflammation associated with delayed-onset muscle soreness (DOMS). This, in turn, helps alleviate muscle soreness and enhance recovery.

However, this anti-inflammatory response can be counterproductive when muscle growth is your goal because inflammation signals muscle repair and growth. By blunting this inflammatory response, cold plunging can potentially interfere with the muscle hypertrophy process and protein synthesis.

If hypertrophy is your goal, the best time to jump in a cold plunge is 4-6 hours after your weight session. If you enjoy a cold plunge after a weight session, reduce the duration (3-5 mins) and ensure the water isn't extremely cold.

Moving beyond muscle gains, cold plunges can be advantageous if you are competing in a tournament or long-distance event over many days to reduce swelling, inflammation, and muscle soreness.

Lastly, consider your personal characteristics. Less intense protocols are recommended for athletes with low body fat and low muscle mass.

Hot Water Immersion involves immersing your body (excluding the head) in warm water above 36°C, typically in one continuous session.

Why do it? Hot Water Immersion aims to relax and relieve muscle tension by increasing blood flow and body temperature. Limiting sessions to around 20 minutes for optimal hot water immersion to maximise relaxation without overexposure. While widely favoured by athletes for its comfort and soothing effects, it's important to avoid hot water immersion if soft tissue injuries are suspected or if the body is already overheated post-exercise.

Contrast Water Therapy proves to be a versatile and effective recovery tool for athletes. By alternating warm and cold immersion into the post-exercise routine, athletes can optimise recovery, reduce muscle soreness, and promote sustained performance gains.

Contrast Water Therapy significantly reduces delayed-onset muscle soreness (DOMS), pain perception reduction, and swelling. It induces vasoconstriction/vasodilation to help eliminate metabolic byproducts (waste) built up in the cell, subsequently supporting overall muscle health.

The recommended protocol for water contrast therapy can vary, and it's essential to consider individual preferences and specific recovery needs. Here's a general guideline:

Water Temperatures:

- Warm Water: Typically, between 38-40°C (100-104°F)
- Cold Water: Typically, between 10-15°C (50-59°F)

Duration:

- Warm Immersion: 3-5 minutes
- Cold Immersion: 1-2 minutes

Number of Cycles: Repeat the warm and cold cycles 3 to 5 times and increase the cycle length if desired.

Order of Immersion: Start with warm water immersion and follow with cold water immersion.

Frequency: CWT sessions can be performed daily, depending on the intensity of the exercise and recovery needs.

Compression Garments or Clothing

Wearing compression sleeves positively affects athletic performance and recovery in specific scenarios. However, the magnitude of these effects is generally small, and the practical relevance should be considered. Some evidence shows that it may contribute to maximal strength and power recovery, joint awareness, reduced muscle swelling and perceived pain, and decreased muscle soreness.

This is a positive list of benefits, and with no downsides observed, except for the cost, these potential effects on recovery should positively influence the subsequent sessions or performance, so they are worth considering.

Pneumatic (air) Leg Compression Boots

Also known as compression therapy, these boots have gained popularity as a recovery tool for athletes. These boots typically consist of inflatable chambers that sequentially apply pressure to different parts of the legs, promoting blood flow and reducing muscle soreness.

The sequential compression action of these boots promotes enhanced blood circulation in the lower extremities, similar to massage. This increased circulation aids in the removal of metabolic byproducts and facilitates the delivery of oxygen and nutrients to muscles. This can lead to reduced muscle soreness and faster recovery.

The intermittent pressure applied by the boots may help reduce swelling and inflammation. This is beneficial in managing the acute effects of exercise-induced trauma and promoting a more comfortable recovery process. The other benefit is they are now readily available at affordable prices, so they can be used in the comfort of your own homes or at training facilities, making them a practical addition to recovery routines.

Massage

Massage is a widely embraced recovery tool with various potential benefits. While the literature presents mixed findings, massage is commonly associated with psychological relief, reduced muscle soreness, and improved flexibility. Applied within 2 hours after exercise, a 20–30 minute massage effectively reduces delayed-onset muscle soreness (DOMS) for up to 96 hours, contributing to improved recovery. It may aid in blood flow, potentially facilitating the removal of metabolic waste products and reducing inflammation.

Athletes often prefer massage for its perceived relaxation benefits. To apply massage effectively, post-exercise, sessions ranging from 15 to 30 minutes are suggested, focusing on major muscle groups. If you don't have access to or can't afford a massage therapist, compression boots or foam rolling can be suitable replacements for massage.

Foam Rolling

Due to the low entry bar, foam rolling is now a popular myofascial release technique for recovery and flexibility. It involves applying pressure to specific points on the body using a foam roller. Research has shown it can alleviate muscle soreness and improve recovery after strenuous exercise. If enough pressure is applied to the muscle and connective tissue, it can help break down adhesions and knots, reducing inflammation and pain. Aim for sessions lasting 5 to 15 minutes. This time frame allows sufficient attention to different muscle groups without overdoing it. Start with the major back and leg muscle groups, focusing on areas prone to tightness. Spend 1-2 minutes on each major muscle group, with additional time on areas of tightness.

Foam rolling can also be done pre-exercise (pre-rolling) and can be an effective strategy for achieving short-term flexibility improvements and potentially reducing DOMS's severity.

Active Recovery

Active recovery requires engaging in low-intensity exercises or activities after intense workouts. It aims to enhance recovery by promoting blood circulation, reducing muscle stiffness, and preventing metabolic byproduct accumulation. Evidence suggests that the appropriate intensity level of active recovery will depend on your sport and fitness levels, but interventions lasting 6-10 minutes consistently demonstrate positive effects on recovery.

Types of Active Recovery:

- Light cardiovascular exercise, e.g., walking, cycling, or swimming.
- Slow controlled breathing exercises
- Low-intensity resistance training, using lighter weights or less volume.
- Yoga or mobility exercises focusing on flexibility, balance, and controlled movements.

Active recovery is no longer just based on performing low-intensity exercises but now includes mindfulness breathing and relaxation techniques. Practising slow, deep breathing after exercise is crucial for aiding the body's recovery by down-regulating your nervous system so the healing process can begin sooner.

How to Implement Active Recovery:

1. Post-Workout Routine: Schedule 10-20 minutes of active recovery following intense workouts. Include a combination of light cardio, slow controlled breathing and stretching exercises.

2. Rest Days: Light recovery sessions can be incorporated after competition or game day or at the end of a hard training week.

While these methods are tried-and-true for enhancing physical recovery, it's essential to recognise the value of complete mental and emotional decompression. Activities that may seem 'unproductive' - like a day at the beach, relaxing with friends, watching a movie, or catching a sports game

- can be just as crucial for reducing allostatic load, the cumulative stress on the body from constant striving and optimisation.

For high performers, these moments of genuine relaxation allow the mind and body to reset, lowering stress hormones and promoting a sense of balance. Embracing these moments without guilt is vital for sustaining peak performance over the long term.

Sleep Challenge - Build Your Foundation For Success

Level 1: Get out of bed at the same time, 6 out of the next 7 days.

Level 1.1: Make that time at or before 6 a.m., 7 a.m. is fine, but only if your chronotype warrants it.

Level 2: Go to bed early enough to allow for an 8-hour window in bed. So, if you are up at 6, you are in bed by 10.

Level 2.1: Stop using all electronic devices 30-60 minutes before bed. Turn off the TV, stop scrolling, stop gaming, etc.

Level 3: Get 10-15 min of sunlight within 30 minutes of waking up. If this is not possible, position yourself in a well-lit area with bright artificial lighting.

Level 4: Download a reliable sleep-tracking app and use it consistently for the next seven nights. Focus on observing your sleep cycles, particularly the amount of deep and REM sleep you're getting each night. This data not only helps you gauge overall sleep quality but can also reveal if you're experiencing frequent awakenings, you may not be aware of, which could be contributing to poor sleep. Understanding these patterns allows you to make informed changes to improve your sleep, health and overall performance.

Level 4.1: Track your pre-bed activities. Note down things like if you exercised that day, ate late, consumed any alcohol or stimulants late in the day, and anything else that may affect your sleep. Most apps allow you to make these notes; if not, you can create one on your phone.

Level 5: Review your sleep scores at the end of the week, identify which nights you slept well or didn't and compare that to the notes on what you did that day and before bed.

Record how you went for the week in the table below, and at the end of the seven days, compare how well you applied the new habits and how this affected your sleep score.

Keep refining your sleep routines and behaviours, and strive for 7-8 hours of quality sleep as often as possible.

Day	Lights off	Wake Up Time	Did I Stop Using Electronic Devices 30-60 mins Before Bed	Sleep Score
1				
2				
3				
4				
5				
6				
7				

Sleep is the foundation on which all other pillars are built!

Pillar 2

Exercise And Stress Management

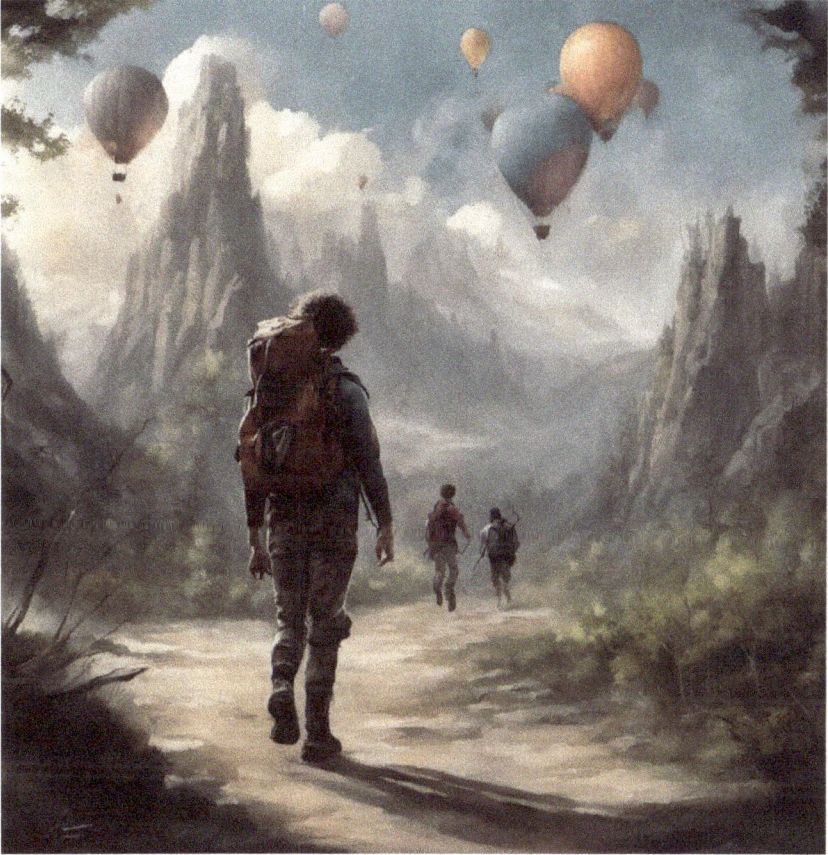

Part 1 - Unlock The Magic Of Movement

Imagine you know where there is a magical fountain containing a liquid that improves your physical, mental, and emotional well-being and helps you live a long and healthy life. All you have to do is walk, ride or run 30 minutes each day to get your daily dose because you can't take any home with you. Would you be willing to do this for such life-changing results?

You might think it's the stuff of fairy tales, but guess what? You have access to these benefits every day. It is not the liquid that provides all those benefits - it's the exercise. Exercise is the turbo boost your life needs, the ultimate elixir of life.

You don't need to be an athlete training 20 hours a week to unleash the magical benefits. Going from doing nothing to being moderately active comes with many fantastic benefits.

The Leap From The Couch: The Power Of Moderate Exercise

Interestingly, the biggest health transformation doesn't require running a marathon or lifting heavy weights six times a week. It's as simple as going from being a couch potato to doing 30 minutes of exercise two to three times a week. Hopefully, this isn't you, but it illustrates the power of exercise.

For instance, a study published in The Lancet in 2016 found that individuals who went from being exercise-phobic to moderately active had a 22% reduction in mortality risk. That's adding an extra decade to your life!

However, don't rest on your laurels just yet. Striving for higher fitness levels can provide additional health benefits and create better habits and performance outcomes. Staying active can be particularly challenging when life gets more demanding due to your commitments and responsibilities. When these times arrive, having well-established exercise habits helps you continue your training because it is an ingrained part of your life. Plus, you know how beneficial your training is to your physical and mental well-being, so even if time is limited, 15 minutes is better than 0 minutes.

Life's Challenges: From Active High School Senior to First-Year Spread

Stepping out of the family nest and living on campus or sharing a house, many young adults face the infamous 'first-year spread.' For most people, exercising or playing sports takes a backseat, food choices diminish, and alcohol consumption increases, all combined with late nights out. This is the perfect recipe for weight gain and establishing unhealthy habits. I'm not saying don't go out, as this is when relationships are formed and memories are made. Just don't let your health and performance suffer at the expense of unnecessary nights out.

The simple solution to combat these challenges is regular exercise. If you are committed to doing cardio or going to the gym throughout the week, you will avoid becoming an unhealthy night creature. Remember, what is good for the heart is good for your brain, so when cognitive development should be in full flight and not your waistline, support it with exercise and sleep.

Landing Your First Serious Job

Statistics suggest a noticeable decline in exercise levels when individuals transition into their first serious job, largely due to increased sedentary behaviour, longer work hours, and the stress of adapting to a new professional environment.

This shift often correlates with a negative health trend, including weight gain, heightened stress levels, and a higher risk for chronic diseases such as diabetes and heart disease. Consequently, the transition into the workforce underscores the importance of finding strategies to integrate physical activity into daily routines to mitigate these health impacts.

Exercise: Your Shield Against Chronic Diseases

Regular exercise is like a shield, protecting you against the onslaught of chronic diseases like heart and lung disease, diabetes, depression and some cancers. Being in the top 20 percentile for your age group typically indicates a high fitness level and better health outcomes, further bolstering your defences. So, you don't need to be elite to get all the benefits of exercise. The most significant health benefits occur by simply going from doing nothing to a moderate amount of exercise.

Why Exercise is Essential for Thriving, Not Just Surviving

The benefits of regular exercise go far beyond physical fitness. Exercise supports brain function, enhances emotional resilience, and regulates essential processes like sleep and appetite. The data is clear: individuals who consistently engage in physical activity don't just live longer - they thrive, enjoying a higher quality of life characterised by better mental health, deeper and more restorative sleep, and sharper cognitive function.

At the heart of exercise's transformative effects are myokines, often called "Hope Molecules." These powerful proteins, released by your muscles during exercise, can cross the blood-brain barrier, directly influencing brain health and function while benefiting your entire body.

Mental Health: Irisin, a myokine released during exercise, crosses the blood-brain barrier and stimulates the production of brain-derived neurotrophic factor (BDNF) in the brain. BDNF promotes neurogenesis (the creation of new neurons), enhances resilience to stress, and may help reduce symptoms of depression and anxiety. By supporting these processes, irisin indirectly improves emotional regulation, sharpens cognitive function, and contributes to long-term brain health and neuroplasticity.

Physical Health: Exercise-induced myokines, such as interleukin-6 (IL-6), are critical in promoting overall physical health. IL-6 released during exercise has anti-inflammatory effects, improves insulin sensitivity, and supports glucose uptake, stabilising blood sugar levels. Additionally, IL-6 promotes fat oxidation, aids energy metabolism and protects against chronic conditions like type 2 diabetes and cardiovascular disease.

Overall Longevity: By mitigating systemic inflammation, optimising metabolic health, and preserving the brain and muscles from age-related decline, myokines ensure that regular exercise not only extends your lifespan but also elevates your quality of life at every stage.

Through the release of myokines, exercise acts as a bridge between movement and holistic health, enhancing mental clarity, physical vitality, and overall well-being.

For most people, the aim should be to rank in the top 20% of physical activity levels for their age group. Achieving this unlocks exercise's profound, life-enhancing benefits, empowering the mind, fortifying the body, and uplifting the spirit. When you move with intention and consistency, the rewards are nothing short of transformative, shaping a healthier, more vibrant life.

How To Know You Are In The Top 20 Percent - Fitness Testing

Each sport, activity, or goal requires different fitness components to be worked on. Each component relates to distinct aspects of your performance, so knowing what you want to achieve is important.

Athletes should be tested and retested across various fitness categories to ensure they are moving in the right direction. However, even if you are not a super serious athlete, I still recommend testing or monitoring the performance or progress of your training routine. It allows you to set a goal and have something to aim at, which can be a great motivator.

One of the many benefits of fitness testing is that it provides direction and keeps you accountable. When I first started writing this book, one of my goals was to row 1 kilometre on a rowing machine in 3 minutes and 30 seconds. As I complete this second edition, I'm proud to share that I've achieved that goal after 9 months of consistent effort. My new goal is to lower that time to 3 minutes and 20 seconds, so perhaps by the time you are reading this, I'll have reached it. And when I do, I'll revise my goals and set a new goal for whatever area I want to progress in next, and on we go.

I also use the rowing machine to complete a 2km time trial to calculate my estimated VO2 Max, the maximum amount of oxygen an individual can use during intense or maximal exercise. This tells me where I rank on the VO2 Max score chart, and I can see if my cardiorespiratory endurance is good, excellent, or elite. Having these performance goals is a great motivator.

Gathering data can be a daily, weekly, or monthly activity. Depending on the level at which you are training and performing, you can make this a regular activity, done at the start and end of a training program, or simply once or twice a year to assess your performance.

When selecting tests, it is important to find a standard test with a set procedure you can follow to implement the same process each time to ensure accurate results. Optimally, find one with normative data (test scores representative of the general population) to compare your results against. By comparing results against other athletes in the same sport, you can see the areas that need improvement, and your training program can be modified accordingly. This way, you know where to focus your energy and your valuable training time can be used more efficiently.

The components of fitness that have well-established tests are:

- cardiovascular endurance or aerobic endurance (VO2 Max)
- anaerobic
- strength
- muscular endurance
- speed
- power
- agility
- flexibility
- balance and coordination

As you can see, there are many components of fitness, so it is essential to focus on the elements that relate to your sports or exercise routine. When it comes to obtaining data, this should also include body composition.

Body composition can provide valuable information about your health and progress, so pick a method or tool, e.g., scale, tape measure, photos, or body scans, and monitor your progress throughout your journey.

The initial testing session provides a snapshot of your current fitness levels or skills, which is used to establish a baseline, and future testing can be compared to this. A starting point is especially important if you are about to embark on a new training program. Subsequent tests should be planned for the end and start of each new training phase. By repeating tests at regular intervals, you can get an idea of the effectiveness of the training program.

The time frame between tests can depend on the availability of time, the costs involved or the phase of training you are in. Depending on these factors, the period between tests may range from two weeks to six months. It usually takes a minimum of 2-6 weeks to see a significant change in any aspect of fitness.

When selecting fitness tests, I recommend choosing tests that require minimal equipment, align with your current fitness level and goals and are easy to implement and repeat.

A great resource that has 300 fitness tests to choose from is Top End Sports. *www.topendsports.com/testing/tests.htm*

One of the most important measurements everyone should know is their VO2 max because it is a powerful metric that goes beyond measuring just athletic prowess. Higher VO2 max scores are associated with a lower risk of cardiovascular diseases, improved metabolic health, and reduced mortality rates. This means a healthier heart, better blood pressure regulation, and more effective management of blood sugar levels.

A higher VO2 max reflects superior cardiovascular health, greater physical fitness, and a better capacity to handle the stressors of physical activity and daily life.

Calculators are available to help translate your results from the different tests into a VO2 max score, allowing you to see where you stand.

The Beep test (20-meter multistage fitness test) is commonly used as a sub-maximal aerobic fitness test and can be used to indicate VO2 max.

If you're into field sports, the 2 km time trial run is a great test to check your aerobic fitness. It's simple yet effective: cover that 2 km distance as fast as possible. Next time you are out on a run or in the gym, see how fast you can cover 2KMs. Here are current records to see how you fare.

2 Kilometre Run Times

	Beginner (Minutes)	Intermediate (Minutes)	Advance (Minutes)	World Record (Minutes)
Women	13.29	9.49	8.38	5.19
Men	11.56	8.25	7.20	4.43

Now, when strength is important, the 1 or 5 Repetition Maximum (1RM) Test is your go-to.

It's how you understand your maximal strength for specific exercises. Knowing this helps customise your training program, ensuring every workout is both safe and effective.

If you're more of a casual fitness enthusiast, think bodyweight exercises. Classics tests like max push-ups and squats aren't just a workout; they are a great way to continually monitor your muscular strength and endurance. Plus, they are easy to implement, adaptable and cater to all fitness levels.

Finally, I want to add functional movement screening. These are specific movement-based tests that help identify movement imbalances and asymmetries. Fixing these imbalances or weaknesses can be done with targeted exercises. Doing this boosts your overall training capacity and significantly lowers the risk of injuries. You may need an experienced coach for these tests, but it is worth doing if you have constant niggling injuries or have acute pain when you lift weights.

A powerful link exists between setting goals, completing fitness tests, and achieving personal success because what gets measured gets managed. So, if you aim to be your best, regularly putting yourself through fitness testing can be the game-changer between reaching your peak or settling for average.

When I work with clients, our journey starts with a conversation to learn about their current activities and goals. Based on that, we will pick the perfect fitness tests to guide the design of the exercise program. They dive into the program for 4-8 weeks, and then we retest. This provides an ongoing progress report and a chance to celebrate wins and fine-tune the plan for even more success. I mention this because appropriate fitness testing should support an effective exercise program.

If you don't have a coach/trainer and need help carrying out tests, get a training partner to assist you so they can help measure and motivate you to get the best results. Then, apply this valuable information to guide what exercises you put into your training program and retest to see if your training produces the desired effects.

So, here's to setting goals, pushing limits, being consistent, and always aiming to be your best.

Part 2 - Move Your Way - There Is No 'One-Size-Fits-All' Exercise Routine

Ultimately, your goals and experience will determine the type and intensity of your training program. You want to find the training routine that is just as unique as you are! This can be hard because, guess what? There's no "one-size-fits-all" in the realm of training programs. So, let's dive into this exciting journey of self-discovery, shall we?

First things first, the basis of an effective fitness routine lies in its sustainability. Finding a training routine or sporting activity you love is like meeting your soulmate and forming a long-lasting relationship. If you would rather pole dance than go to the gym, then by all means, dance like nobody's watching! Or, if you're constrained by time and can't hit the gym, no worries! Find a workout that requires minimal equipment and can be done at home.

Remember, the best type of exercise is the one you will do regularly, so be adventurous and experiment until you find your match. Here are some guidelines to help you design your exercise program.

As much as individuality is the key, there are guidelines worth considering. Well-established recommendations for cardiovascular, resistance, and flexibility training ensure that the minimum is done to maintain overall well-being. However, if you have specific fitness goals, you probably need to improve on these guidelines, but we will get to that later.

Weekly Recommended Physical Activity Levels For Each Fitness Category

Cardiovascular Fitness

Frequency: Aim for 150-180 minutes or 3 to 5 sessions of moderate-intensity steady-state aerobic exercise weekly. If you want to improve your peak aerobic threshold, 30 - 60 minutes or 1 -2 sessions of vigorous-intensity exercise per week. These are high-intensity intervals or repeated sprints for peak performance.

Type: Include activities like walking, running, cycling, swimming, or rowing.

Intensity: Zone 2 - Low to moderate (60-70% of max heart rate). You'll still feel relatively comfortable, and you should be able to sustain this level of exercise for extended periods of time.

Zone 3 - Moderate (70-80% Max HR). You can just maintain a conversation, but it will take a bit more effort, and you will be more focused on performing the activity.

Zone 4 - Hard (80-90% Max HR). Shorter efforts will make you acutely aware that you're pushing your limits and working close to your maximum capacity. You are only focused on the job at hand.

Zone 5 - Maximum (90-100% of Max HR). This is an all-out effort level, sustainable only for short bursts. When you're in Zone 5, you're at your absolute limits.

Deep Dive Into Zone 2 Training: Your training intensity is very important for improving cardiovascular endurance and mitochondrial function. When training in zone 2, the body predominantly uses fat as a fuel source, improving fat oxidation and lactate threshold, leading to enhanced cardiovascular performance.

Mitochondria are the powerhouses of your cells, responsible for producing energy. Training in zone 2 stimulates mitochondrial biogenesis - the creation of new mitochondria. More and better-performing mitochondria allow your body to produce more energy efficiently, which is vital for sustained endurance efforts.

Improving the lactate threshold will increase the point at which lactate accumulates in the blood faster than it can be cleared. Training in zone 2 helps increase the efficiency of your mitochondria, which delays the point at which lactate begins to accumulate. Over time, this can raise your lactate threshold, allowing you to maintain a higher intensity for longer periods without fatigue.

What happens when we exceed our lactate threshold? When you go beyond your lactate threshold (usually in zone 4 or higher), lactate accumulates rapidly in the blood. Contrary to common belief, lactate itself does not cause acidosis; rather, it is associated with an increase in hydrogen ions (H^+) that lower the pH of the blood, contributing to acidosis and the burning sensation in muscles. This accumulation eventually leads to fatigue and a drop in performance.

However, by developing more and better-performing mitochondria, your muscles can produce more energy aerobically, delaying the accumulation of lactate and hydrogen ions and enhancing your ability to sustain higher efforts for longer periods.

Having efficient mitochondria also increases your body's capacity to oxidise fat, which is particularly beneficial for endurance athletes, as fat is a long-lasting energy source. Improved mitochondrial function means your muscles can sustain higher workloads with less reliance on anaerobic energy systems, reducing fatigue and allowing you to maintain a higher intensity for longer. Focusing on zone 2 training lays the groundwork for improved cardiovascular endurance, enhanced mitochondrial function, and a higher lactate threshold. All key elements for long-term athletic performance and sustained work capacity.

In practice, the heart rate zone you work in must be tailored to your fitness levels. Someone well-trained might see mitochondrial benefits at a slightly higher heart rate (zone 3), while less-trained individuals might need to stay lower (in zone 2) to achieve similar results without overloading their system. The exact zone or heart rate that elicits mitochondrial improvements can vary, so personalising training zones based on testing and individual response is key.

Let's use a more accurate formula for calculating your estimated max heart rate than the old 220 - age.

Predicted Max Heart Rate = $208 - (0.7 \times age)$

Predicted max heart rate for a 25-year-old: $208 - (0.7 \times 25) = 190.5$ BPM

Zone	% of Max Heart Rate	Heart Rate (BPM)	Training Goal
1 Very Light	50-60%	95 - 114	Warm-up and recovery
2 Light	61-70%	114 -133	Base-level aerobic activities
3 Moderate	71-80%	133 - 152	Aerobic endurance events
4 Hard	81-90%	152 - 171	Anaerobic short-distance/ field sports
5 Maximal	91-100%	171 - 190	Short Burst Speed Training

Flexibility and Mobility

Frequency: For optimal results, aim to incorporate flexibility and mobility work into your routine at least 2-3 days per week. Consistency is key to improving your range of motion and reducing the risk of injury. This can be done as part of your warm-up, cool-down, or dedicated session.

Incorporate flexibility and mobility work into your daily routine. For example, if you're watching TV at the end of the day, use that time to get on the floor with a foam roller or a trigger point massage ball. Focus on areas that feel tight or have a limited range of motion. Lying on the ground is also an excellent opportunity to perform static stretches or work on hip and thoracic mobility.

What types of stretching should you do?

Static Stretching involves holding a stretch in a fixed position. It is most effective post-workout and should be avoided before training or a game, as dynamic stretching is more effective in the warm-up. It helps reduce muscle stiffness, promotes muscle length, and improves range of motion.

Dynamic Stretching involves moving parts of your body through a full range of motion, such as leg swings and bodyweight squats. It is best done before a workout to increase blood flow and joint lubrication to improve overall mobility. Choose warm-up movements that mirror the exercises you are about to perform in the body of the session.

Foam Rolling (Self-Myofascial Release): This technique uses a foam roller to release muscle tightness and trigger points. Foam rolling can be done before or after workouts to enhance mobility, reduce muscle soreness, and improve overall flexibility.

If you want a more structured approach, Yoga and Pilates are excellent for improving flexibility and mobility.

Strength or Resistance Training

Frequency: Resistance training should be performed 3-4 days a week, covering all major muscle groups to avoid imbalances. If you are advanced, 4-6 sessions a week may be appropriate.

Type: This will depend on your sport and goal. For all you athletes out there, don't try to mimic the exact movements of your sport in the gym with weights. This can lead to a breakdown in the correct technique and movement pattern of that skill.

To build the best body for your sport, follow a structured exercise program focusing on strength and conditioning. Many variables must be considered when designing an exercise program, and over the next few pages, I have outlined the overarching principles of an effective program.

Intensity: The table below outlines the recommended parameters for different training goals. Aim to train all major muscle groups three or more days a week, completing 4-6 exercises per session. If you are an experienced athlete, you should aim for 18-20 working sets per major muscle group each week.

Training Goal	Sets	Reps	Intensity	Rest
Hypertrophy (building muscle)	3-6	6-12	65-85% 1RM	30-90 sec
Strength	2-6	1-6	80-100% 1RM	2-5 min
Power	3-5	1-5	75-95% 1RM	2-5 min
Endurance	2-4	12-20+	50-67% 1RM	30-60sec
Weight Loss	2-4	12-20+	50-75% 1RM	30-60sec

Here is an example of a weekly training program: a 3-day whole-body program that works with existing activities.

Day 1: Full Body Workout

Warm-Up - 5 Min walk/ride/rowing machine		
Warm-up movements/dynamic stretches - Jumping jacks, bodyweight squats, leg swings, arm circles	20 sec each x 2 rounds	
Exercise	**Sets x Reps**	**Rest (seconds)**
Squats (Back or Goblet)	3 x 12	60-90
Walking lunges	3 x 20 steps	60-90
Lat Pulldown	3 x 12	60-90
Seated Row Machine	3 x 12	60-90
Plank	3 x 30sec	30-60
Cool Down - 5 min walk. Static stretches - quads, hamstrings, back, shoulders		

Day 2: Sports/event-specific training.

Day 3: Full Body Workout

Warm-Up - 5 mins walk/ride/x-trainer		
Warm-up movement/dynamic stretches - Step-ups, leg swings, hip circles, RB pull-apart	20 sec each x 2 rounds	
Exercise	**Sets x Reps**	**Rest (seconds)**
Deadlifts	3 x 12	60-90
Bench Press (Barbell or Dumbbell)	3 x 12	60-90
Single Leg High Step-Ups	3 x 12	60-90
Arnold Shoulder Press	3 x 12	60-90
DB Pec Flys	3 x 12	30-60
Cool Down - 5-10 mins walk/ride. Static Stretches - lower back, glutes, chest		

Day 4: Sport/event-specific training or light active recovery

Day 5: Full Body Workout

Warm-Up - 5 mins walk/ride/x-trainer		
Warm-up movement/dynamic stretches - Bodyweight squat, arm circles, leg swings, hip circles		20 sec each x 2 rounds
Exercise	**Sets x Reps**	**Rest (seconds)**
Box Jumps	3 x 10	60-90
Sled Push (up and back)	3 x 10-15m	60-90
Leg Press	3 x 10	60-90
Chin up and Pull Ups (2 sets of each)	4 x 8	60-90
Lying Bicycle Crunch	3 x 20	30-60
Cool Down - 5 min walk/ride/x-trainer Static Stretches - Hip Flexors, Lower back, glute and hamstring stretches		

Day 6: Perform your chosen sport or event.

Day 7: Active rest - walk/jog, ride, swim and stretch.

Methods To Progress or Regress Your Training

Regressing (Easier)	Variable To Change	Progressing (Harder)
Lighter	**Load (weight)**	Heavier
Fewer	**Repetitions**	More
More	**Rest**	Less
Reduced ROM	**Range of motion (ROM)**	Increase ROM
Static (stationary)	**Complexity of Movement**	Dynamic
Wider base of support or increase points of contact	**Base of Support (stability)**	Decrease the base of support or fewer points of contact
Slower (isometric or static)	**Speed Of Movement**	Faster/Explosive (plyometric/ballistic)

Common Exercise Progression and Regressions

Regression			Gold Standard	Progression		
Level 3	Level 2	Level 1		Level 1	Level 2	Level 3
Box Squat	Bodyweight Squat	Goblet	**Barbell Back Squat**	Front Squat	Overhead Squat	Box Jumps
Seated Chest Press	Push-up	Narrow Grip Bench Press	**Bench Press**	Dumbbell Bench Press	Incline Bench Press	Eccentric/ Banded Bench Press
Dumbbell Deadlift	Rack Deadlifts	Sumo Deadlift	**Barbell Deadlift**	Snatch Grip Deadlift	Deficit Deadlift	Chain or Banded Deadlift
Seated Row	DB 1-arm Bent-Over Row	Underhand grip BB Bent-Over Row	**Barbell Bent-Over Row**	Chest Supported DB Row	Pendlay Barbell Row	Chin Ups or Pull Ups

The Importance of Periodisation in Your Training Program

Many exercise principles can be applied to a training program, but if you're unsure how to progress and achieve better results, approach it as you would learning any new skill: seek guidance from someone knowledgeable and start by mastering the fundamentals. Be honest about your current skill level and physical abilities and adopt a long-term perspective for continual improvements. A well-structured program tailored to your goals and abilities is essential for lasting success.

A periodised training program is a proven system for designing and progressing your training in a systematic and strategic way. Once you have clearly outlined your goals, identify the variables in your training, such as intensity, volume, frequency, and exercise selection, and structure your plan to align with your timeline and objectives.

What is Periodisation?

Periodisation is a method of varying key training components over specific time frames to achieve peak performance. Unlike a static, one-size-fits-all approach, periodisation involves adjusting intensity, volume, and frequency to ensure optimal progress while avoiding plateaus or overtraining. For example:

- When intensity increases (e.g., heavier weights), volume (e.g., total sets or reps) may need to decrease.

- During high-volume phases, intensity and frequency might be adjusted to prevent overtraining.

This structured approach enables you to build strength, endurance, or skill systematically, ensuring you are at your best when it matters most.

Phases of Periodisation

A periodised program is often divided into distinct phases, each with a specific purpose:

1. **Hypertrophy (Muscle Growth):** Focuses on higher volume and moderate intensity to build muscle size and endurance.

    - Example: 10–12 reps with moderate weights and shorter rest periods for 8 weeks.

2. **Strength:** Lower reps and higher loads to increase maximal force production.

    - Example: 3–6 reps with heavy weights and longer rest periods for 4 weeks.

3. **Skill or Competition Preparation:** Fine-tune performance by incorporating sport-specific movements, higher intensity, or peaking strategies.

    - Example: Explosive, high-intensity training that converts the strength and size you have developed to improve your sport specific skills or athletic ability.

4. **Recovery or Deloading:** Allows the body and nervous system to recover and adapt, reducing injury risk and preventing burnout.

- Example: Lower intensity or active recovery sessions with lighter weights or reduced volume.

Benefits of Periodisation

Incorporating periodisation into your routine ensures your training remains:

- **Dynamic and Effective:** By cycling through different phases, you avoid monotony and ensure progressive overload.

- **Adaptable to Goals:** Allows adjustments as your goals or physical condition evolve.

- **Injury-Minimising:** Systematic changes in volume and intensity reduce overuse injuries and improve recovery.

- **Performance-Optimising:** Prepares you to peak at the right time, whether for competition or personal milestones.

Practical Application

Periodisation doesn't need to be overly complicated. Start with simple adjustments based on your timeline and goals:

- If reps increase, reduce the load.

- When volume is high, keep intensity moderate level.

- As a competition or milestone approaches, shift focus to skill execution and peaking.

The exact mix of variables depends on your sport, activity, or desired outcome. For example, an endurance athlete may prioritise high-volume aerobic training early in the cycle, tapering to focus on speed and race-specific efforts closer to the event.

Why Periodisation Matters

Periodising your training ensures a structured path to continual improvement while keeping your program engaging and sustainable. It allows you to maximise performance, reduce injury risk, and maintain enthusiasm for your workouts. Whether you're an athlete preparing for competition or simply striving for personal fitness goals, periodisation is your roadmap to peak performance and long-term success.

Periodisation at work, with the different terminology used across various sports.

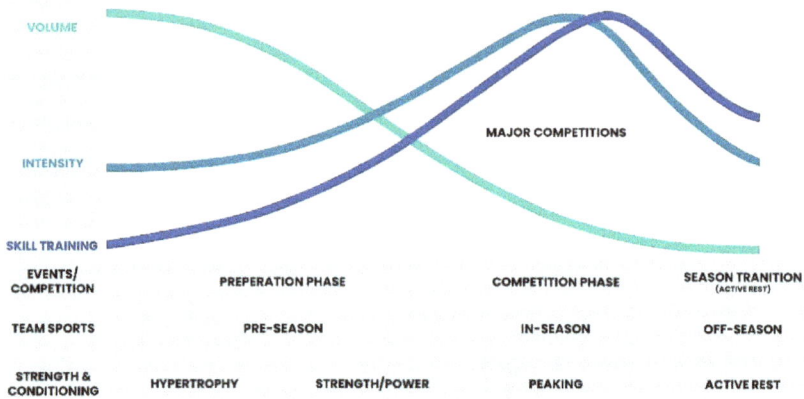

	PREPERATION PHASE		COMPETITION PHASE	SEASON TRANITION (ACTIVE REST)
EVENTS/ COMPETITION				
TEAM SPORTS	PRE-SEASON		IN-SEASON	OFF-SEASON
STRENGTH & CONDITIONING	HYPERTROPHY	STRENGTH/POWER	PEAKING	ACTIVE REST

The Tale Of Progression: Slow and Steady Wins The Race

Remember the story of the tortoise and the hare? That lesson applies perfectly to building long-term success in any training program. Progress isn't about how fast you can go - it's about steady and consistent improvement.

When starting a new program, resist the temptation to compare yourself to others or rush into executing complex skills at the same level as someone with years of experience.

Instead, focus on mastering the fundamentals. Be honest about your current capabilities, and commit to gradual, incremental improvements. Each small step forward builds a strong foundation for long-term progress, minimising the risk of injury and setbacks.

Steady, continual progress helps you reach your goals more sustainably and builds confidence and resilience along the way. Trust the process, and your body and mind will thank you.

The Perils Of Missing Workouts: Don't Break The Chain

Missing a workout occasionally is no biggie, but don't make a habit of it! Remember, consistency is key. So, even if you only squeeze in a 15-minute workout, it's better than nothing. Because every time you show up for yourself, you're reinforcing that you are a high performer and making a vote for the person you want to be.

Skipping one session might not feel like a big deal, but before you know it, you have missed an entire week. And guess what? You're not only losing progress but also getting good at not showing up, and that's a habit you definitely don't want to be good at!

The Psychological Power Of Sticking To A Training Program

Physical training isn't just about getting stronger or faster; it also strengthens your mind. Those moments when you push through, even when you don't want to, build resilience and discipline. We all have days when we don't want to train, but overcoming those voices in your head saying you are too tired or it's too hot or cold outside is where you build mental strength and discipline.

Motivation is fleeting, but discipline is there when things are hard. Regardless of how you feel, you will still show up and vote for the person you want to be. Remember, every challenge you overcome in your training makes the everyday stressors of life seem easier to manage. Choosing to do hard things daily hardens your mind against feeling weak, vulnerable and underprepared in times of adversity. Getting comfortable with being uncomfortable serves you in all areas of life.

Here are 5 strategies to optimise your progress, prevent injuries, and align the exercises with your goals.

Josh's Performance Tips

Prioritise Movement Quality: I can't emphasise the importance of proper form and technique when training with weights. Movement quality maximises muscle engagement and reduces the risk of injuries. When introducing new exercises, learn the correct movement patterns, ensuring that each repetition is performed correctly. Master the movement pattern before adding weight or advancing the exercise. Getting injured means, you are not training and losing progress. Leave your ego at the door and train with longevity in mind.

Individualise Your Approach: Your anatomy, mobility, and goals are unique. So, you need to personalise your approach to training, considering factors such as experience, strengths, weaknesses/limitations and desired outcomes. Tailor exercises to suit your specific needs or sport for a more effective and sustainable training experience. Don't follow the crowd if you want a specific outcome.

Periodise Your Training: This is where training is structured into different phases, which is especially important if you are an athlete. Even changing or modifying your gym program every 6-8 weeks is a basic form of periodisation. This approach helps prevent plateaus, reduces the risk of overtraining, and keeps the training stimulus challenging. Your training program should cycle through higher intensity, volume, load and recovery phases to optimise performance and long-term progress.

Focus On Recovery and Regeneration: Don't underestimate the significance of including recovery in the overall training equation. Quality sleep, proper nutrition, and active recovery techniques are crucial in enhancing performance and preventing burnout. This means taking a holistic approach to health that extends beyond the gym.

Set Clear and Realistic Goals: High performers need to establish clear, measurable, and realistic goals. Whether you want to increase strength, build muscle, improve endurance, or develop sport-specific skills, having a clear vision and well-defined goal provides direction and motivation. Don't forget to review and adjust goals when necessary.

Your fitness routine will look different depending on your chosen sport or activity. Some of you reading this will already have a well-established gym or training routine, but please don't forget to incorporate the other areas of fitness required to stay injury-free and at your peak.

So, What's the Takeaway?

Adherence is Key! Whether you prefer weightlifting, cycling, yoga, or another form of exercise, the most important factor is finding an activity you genuinely enjoy. It's not about conforming to a standard; it's about embracing what makes you feel alive and gives you purpose. After all, the most effective workout is the one you'll stick with over time.

If you're serious about staying on track, progressing consistently, and optimising your performance, consider hiring a trainer. A good coach is worth their weight in gold, providing tailored guidance, support, and accountability.

To help you on your high-performance journey, here are a few of the best-rated apps across iOS and Android:

1. **Future** (Personalised Weightlifting App): This app offers tailored workout programs created by real trainers who provide feedback, accountability, and adjustments based on your progress.

2. **Shred App** (Weightlifting App for Home Gyms): Designed for those working out at home, offering guided workouts tailored to the equipment you have on hand.

3. **Caliber** (Weightlifting App with Nutrition Coaching): Combines data-driven training with nutrition coaching, making it ideal for those seeking both workout guidance and dietary support.

4. **ClassPass** (Weightlifting App for Classes): Perfect for those who enjoy the group fitness environment, ClassPass gives access to a wide range of virtual and in-person classes.

5. **Strong** (Tracker App for Weightlifting): This app provides a simple and intuitive way to log workouts, track progress, and monitor strength gains over time, ideal for dedicated lifters.

6. **RepCount** (Free Weightlifting App): This is a no-cost option that offers effective tracking features, including sets, reps, and weight logs, with an easy-to-use interface.

7. **JEFIT** (Weightlifting App for Beginners): This app features an extensive exercise database and beginner-friendly workout plans, making it ideal for those new to strength training.

Choose the app that best aligns with your goals, input your fitness level, and let it guide you toward a more rewarding routine. Remember, progress over perfection is the goal - enjoy the journey, stay consistent, and build lasting habits!

"It is the work done in the unseen hours, that separates the great from the good."

Part 3 - Stress - Friend Or Foe?

Meet Stress: Your Unexpected Ally and Occasional Foe

What if I told you that stress could be your friend? Yes, you read that right. It's like that friend who loves to party but doesn't know when to stop. They can be fun and motivating initially but annoying and detrimental when they get too drunk and won't go home. Let's delve into the complexities of this relationship and learn how stress can be both a hero and a villain in our lives.

A Tale of Two Stresses

Imagine you're on a camping trip and encounter a big, hungry grizzly bear. Your heart starts to race, blood pressure increases, and your body prepares for action by releasing adrenaline and cortisol. That's stress in a nutshell. It's your body's way of saying, "Hey, we've got a problem here, let's deal with it." This acute stress response can be quite the lifesaver in such situations.

But what happens when that bear follows you home, starts hanging out in your backyard, and is always watching you, ready to take you out? That's chronic stress. It's like having a wild animal stalking you 24/7. Not exactly a recipe for relaxation.

Acute Stress: The Unsung Hero

Let's take a moment to appreciate the benefits of acute stress. It sharpens focus, mobilises energy, and heightens attentional capacity, enabling improved performance in tasks that demand concentration and quick decision-making. This surge in arousal can also amplify motivation and drive, fostering greater productivity and efficiency in achieving goals.

This fight-or-flight is designed to increase heart rate, blood pressure, and energy availability to enhance our physical capabilities and situational awareness for short periods to overcome adversity and danger. However, it is much safer in our modern world than 1000 years ago, and we more commonly use acute stress to help us meet deadlines, deal with accidents, or perform our best on the sports field. A little bit of stress can help you focus and get you moving. For most people, it produces positive outcomes.

However, there will be times when acute stress causes emotional discomfort, anxiety, and irritability, which can negatively impact performance and well-being. Hence, it is important to recognise when you are stressed, as this will allow you to reframe how you deal with the situation and overcome challenges. In the performance arena, preparation is the key to overcoming self-doubt and using stress to your advantage.

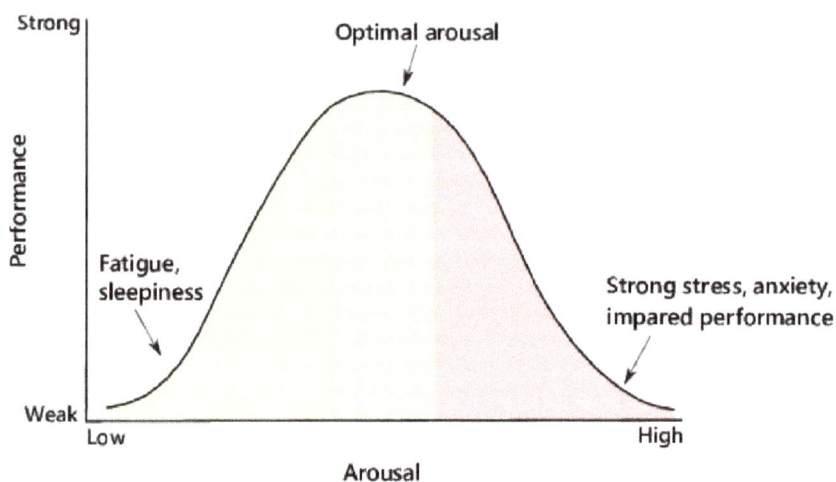

The Yerkes-Dodson Law describes the relationship between arousal (or stress) and performance. The law suggests there is an optimal level of arousal for a given task, but too little or too much can impede performance. Like Goldilocks, applying the concept of "just the right amount" is how to approach arousal when you need to perform at your best.

Here's a breakdown of the key concepts:

Low Arousal (Left Side of the Curve): When arousal is low, performance will likely be low. This is because individuals may lack the motivation and focus to engage effectively in the task. A certain baseline level of arousal is needed for optimal focus and performance.

Optimal Arousal (Peak of the curve): A moderate level of arousal (stress) goes a long way. It's manageable, motivational, and performance-enhancing. Your heart rate is up but steady, and you feel a sense of clarity and alertness. Your brain and body are all fired up. This is an optimal level of arousal where performance is maximised. This sweet spot is where individuals are sufficiently stimulated and motivated, enhancing focus, attention, and output in completing tasks.

High Arousal (Right Side of the Curve): In these situations, stress and anxiety are ramping up to an unmanageable level. Your heart is beating faster, and your hands are shaky, which is unsettling, distracting, and even nerve-wracking. Performance starts to decline as arousal increases beyond the optimal point. Too much stress or arousal can decrease the ability to concentrate and block out the external environment, causing overwhelm and suboptimal performance.

Identifying what stresses you out and detracts from you showing up at your best is a game changer. Techniques such as positive self-talk, visualisation, controlled breathing, and progressive muscle relaxation can all be used to calm the nervous system.

In my experience, being underprepared is a surefire way to raise stress levels to 10 out of 10, and positive self-talk or visualisation will not help much. Your brain knows what you are capable of and will not be fooled by false bravado. Being prepared brings confidence and, combined with the right behaviours, will produce the optimal level of arousal for you to perform at your best in tasks ranging from exams to athletic competitions.

I will share a personal story to see this concept in action: I'm competing in the Hervey Bay men's A-grade hockey grand finale, one of my sporting career's most intense and exhilarating moments. The game was a relentless battle, 70 minutes of full-throttle play that ended in a 2-2 deadlock. We went into overtime, 5 minutes each way, but with still no winner after overtime, we faced the high-stakes pressure of penalty shootouts.

It is you against the goalkeeper, and all you have to do is flick the ball past the keeper into the goal. Flicking the ball is usually a simple skill, but the pressure becomes immense when the game is on the line. It was the best out of five shots for each team, and it was decided that I would go last from our team. After nine shots, it came down to the last shot, and now it was my turn.

The opposition was up by a goal, so the situation was crystal clear: If I miss, they win the premiership. These moments are rare in your sporting career, and I always dreamed about being the game-winner when my team needed me, but now everything came down to one shot.

As I walked out to take the shot, I felt the weight of the moment, but instead of letting it overwhelm me, I used the pressure to my advantage. The stress heightened my senses, allowing me to zone out the noise and focus solely on the task - go out there and put the ball into the back of the net!

I began visualising where I wanted the ball to go, studying the goalie's eyes and body movements. When the umpire asked if we were ready, I felt calm and focused - a result of harnessing the stress to become hyper-focused.

The whistle blew. I watched the goalie shift his weight to his left foot, giving me the split-second confirmation I needed. As the goalie pushed off to cover his right side, I sent the ball flying into the top left corner of the net. The crowd went wild because this epic battle wasn't over yet.

The stakes went even higher as the match entered sudden death; the next missed shot would determine the victor. The opposing team's captain was up next, a player of undeniable skill. Every eye was locked on him as he prepared to shoot. The tension was palpable; the crowd hushed when the whistle blew for him to shoot, and he sent his shot wide. We realised we had secured the victory at that moment, and the celebrations began.

There is a caveat here. I knew that trusting my training was key. All those hours spent hitting and flicking balls had prepared me for this moment. I didn't need to second-guess myself; I knew I had the skills, and I just had to execute. When you're in a high-pressure situation, you can't fake confidence with a bit of positive self-talk. If you fake it, you won't make it. You must genuinely trust your abilities, built through consistent training and preparation. Then, you can use the pressure of the situation to lift you up and do great things.

Understanding that acute stress can actually enhance performance is essential. The key to leveraging it effectively lies in discovering your optimal stress zone and developing strategies to manage overwhelming situations, which we will touch on soon.

Chronic Stress: The Unwanted Houseguest

Chronic stress is like that houseguest who overstays their welcome and starts to take over your house. At first, their presence might seem manageable, even necessary in a crisis. But as time goes on, they begin to drain your energy (constantly elevated cortisol), disrupt your daily routines (interfere with sleep), and create long-term turmoil (emotional and physical health issues). Just as you would take decisive action to reclaim your home, it's essential to confront and manage chronic stress before it takes an irreversible toll on your health and well-being.

The Biochemical Storm

When you encounter stress, your body launches into action, releasing a surge of hormones like cortisol and adrenaline. This response perfectly suits short-term challenges, preparing you to confront or escape this situation. However, when stress becomes a constant presence, this biochemical storm never fully dissipates, leading to a cascade of health issues.

Cortisol's Role

Often referred to as the "stress hormone," cortisol is released by your adrenal glands in response to stress. It signals the liver to release glucose into the bloodstream, providing a quick energy boost to tackle immediate threats. While this is useful in the short term, chronic stress keeps your body in a perpetual state of high alert. The constant release of glucose can eventually lead to insulin resistance, a precursor to type 2 diabetes and disrupt your body's ability to maintain stable blood sugar levels and metabolise fats.

Adrenaline's Impact

Adrenaline (epinephrine in the USA), another key player in the stress response, is released from the adrenal medulla. Adrenaline increases your heart rate and blood pressure, preparing you for immediate action. But when this response is continuous, it leads to chronically elevated blood pressure, which can damage your cardiovascular system over time.

In discussions of chronic stress, the term "adrenal fatigue" often surfaces. Adrenal fatigue is the idea that people who are under long-term mental, emotional, or physical stress can lead to overuse and eventual burnout of the adrenal glands. This results in symptoms like fatigue, body aches, trouble sleeping, and the need for stimulants like caffeine to get through the day. However, it's important to note that adrenal fatigue is not a recognised medical diagnosis.

The Endocrine Society and other leading health organisations do not acknowledge adrenal fatigue as a legitimate disease. Instead, what is often described as adrenal fatigue may actually be a symptom of other underlying conditions, such as chronic fatigue syndrome, depression, hypothyroidism or sleep apnea. In some cases, these symptoms may indicate adrenal insufficiency, known as Addison's disease, a medical condition where the adrenal glands do not produce sufficient hormones due to damage or dysfunction.

Sleep Disruption

One of chronic stress's most insidious effects is its impact on sleep. Stress hormones interfere with your body's natural circadian rhythms, making it difficult to fall or stay asleep. Over time, this lack of restorative sleep exacerbates stress, creating a vicious cycle of being too stressed to sleep and too sleep-deprived to manage stress effectively.

Behavioural Change

In response to chronic stress, your behaviour may also shift in ways that perpetuate the problem. You might turn to coping mechanisms like overeating, withdrawing from social interactions, or increasing your reliance on substances like alcohol or caffeine. While these behaviours may offer temporary relief, they often introduce new stressors - poor diet, not sleeping, isolation, and substance dependency - that further entrench the cycle of stress.

Why You Should Show Chronic Stress the Door

When stress becomes a constant presence, it can lead to what scientists call an 'allostatic load' - a constant force on your body. It's like having a heavy backpack that you can't take off. Over time, it will pull you down.

But don't despair! Just as you can learn to juggle oranges, play a guitar, and drive a car, you can learn to manage stress.

In challenging situations, there's a popular saying: control the controllables. It's simple advice that may help ease the burden you are feeling, but let's go one step better and provide more context you can apply to help you focus your energy and attention. I want to introduce you to the Circle of Concern and Circle of Influence. This great framework will help you gain clarity, keep anxiety in check, and focus your efforts on areas you can truly impact, supporting positive momentum in your life.

The Circle of Concern/Circle of Influence

A great way to become more self-aware and in control of your life's stresses is to look at where you are focusing your attention and energy. A great tool you can use, which I learned in the 7 Habits of Highly Successful People, is the "Circle of Concern/Circle of Influence."

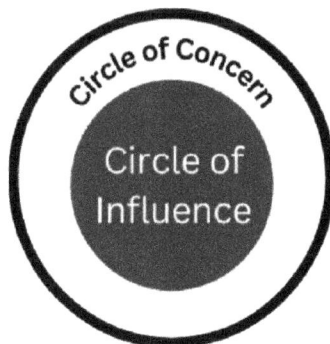

Your Circle of Concern includes everything you're worried about but have little or no control over. These might be global issues like international politics, climate change, or economic downturns. They could also involve societal trends, such as the rise of technology replacing jobs or cultural shifts you feel uneasy about. Personal concerns might include other people's opinions of you, what a co-worker did or didn't do or the actions of distant acquaintances.

While it's natural to care about these matters, it's important to recognise that investing too much energy in them is counterproductive to achieving your goals and living a happy and fulfilling life. For example, constantly stressing over news headlines, fretting about the outcome of an election in another country, or worrying about the end of days for humanity leads to unnecessary anxiety. It's akin to trying to change the weather by worrying about it - a drain on your energy with no tangible benefit. By acknowledging these concerns but choosing to focus your efforts elsewhere, you can reduce stress and direct your energy toward areas where you can actually make a difference.

Our **Circle of Influence** includes the things we can do something about. These are the areas we have direct control over, such as our attitudes, behaviours, and actions. The extent of your influence will relate to your position in your family, team, organisation, community or country. The company's CEO will have greater influence over the direction of the company than the workers on the ground. So what does this tell you? Focus on your attitude and actions needed to increase your circle of influence.

Proactive high performers focus their efforts in their circle of influence and work on things they can do something about. Your mental and emotional energy is not endless, so ignore the outside noise and get busy doing things you can influence – this will enable you to make effective changes. If you do this, your circle of influence starts to increase – others will see you as an effective person, increasing your ability to effect change.

Reactive low performers focus their attention on the Circle of Concern. They get wrapped up in things like their sports team losing, problems with the government, a reality TV show, American politics, and what their colleagues said at work, all circumstances over which they have little influence. Generally, this leads to negative attitudes, reactive language, and increased feelings of helplessness and victimisation.

Negative energy creates unnecessary anxiety and stress while neglecting the things they could do something about. By identifying and focusing on what you can control, you channel your energy into productive actions, leading to greater satisfaction and success.

This proactive approach improves your immediate environment and gradually expands your influence over time. For instance, by consistently applying effort to improve your skills and performance at work or training, you may influence larger company decisions, get selected for the team you want to play in or be delegated leadership responsibilities.

Remember, the more time you spend worrying about things in your circle of concern, the worse your feelings of helplessness and anxiety will become. Focus on the things you can control, and your circle of influence will grow. This is how you become an effective high performer.

The prayer from Alcoholics Anonymous sums it up perfectly.

"Lord, give me the courage to change the things which can and ought to be changed, the serenity to accept the things which cannot be changed, and the wisdom to know the difference."

Strategies To Kick Stress To The Curb

The following proven stress-busting strategies can make a real difference in your life. Think of them as tools in your stress management toolkit - some will resonate deeply, while others may not suit you as well. Remember, like any new habit, these techniques require consistency to unlock their full benefits, so commit to the ones that work best for you.

Having multiple go-to strategies is also helpful, as each can be useful in different situations. Let's start with daily strategies to manage stress holistically, giving you a well-rounded approach to staying grounded and resilient. Some of these strategies have been discussed earlier in the book, but I will highlight them again in relation to stress management.

Daily Stress-Beating Strategies

Mindfulness or Guided Meditation

I recommend starting with guided meditation, which involves an instructor or a pre-recorded voice guiding you through a meditation session. When you start meditating, it can be frustrating, but just like any new habit, repetition and consistency are key. This form of meditation is designed to promote heightened self-awareness and to be present in the current moment. Learning to focus and catching negative thoughts that don't serve you can cultivate a clear mind and reduce stress.

Studies conducted by Dr. Amishi Jha with active-duty members of the United States military, specifically from the U.S. Army, demonstrated measurable improvements in participants' attention, focus, and resilience. The research revealed that practicing mindfulness for as little as twelve minutes, five days a week, could lead to significant cognitive benefits, even amidst the high-stress demands of military life. These improvements were particularly notable in enhancing working memory and reducing stress.

Dr. Jha's work underscores that it doesn't take long to see the benefits of mindfulness practice. However, just like learning any new skill or behaviour, it's crucial to start slowly and avoid overwhelming yourself with overly long or demanding sessions. The goal is consistency over time, allowing the positive effects to build gradually while staying realistic about what fits into your routine. Sitting still, focusing on your breath and observing your thoughts is harder than you think. However, if guys in the military can meditate for 12 minutes and gain the benefits, so can you.

One of the worst causes of stress in your life will be your thoughts, so developing the ability to catch yourself when ruminating on negative thoughts is a game changer. Identifying and stopping that loop-of-doom thought pattern will allow you to regain control of your thoughts and turn that stress response off.

This is so important because your body does not know the difference between the actual experience and the memory of that experience replaying in your mind. Ruminating evokes the same emotional and subsequent physiological response as if you were still dealing with the experience that occurred a day, week, or a year ago.

Simply thinking about what happened will instruct your body to produce stress-related hormones that prepare you to deal with the situation at hand. But they are not needed because you are sitting at your desk or lying in bed, and this rumination will only lead to poor physical and mental health. That is why learning to be mindful of your thoughts is one of the best skills you can develop.

Breathwork

Whim Hoff has made breathwork popular over the past decade, and it has become one of my daily habits. It is a breathing technique that involves intentional and rhythmic deep breathing followed by a period of holding your breath. There are many forms of breathwork, so I recommend starting with guided beginner sessions of 10-15 minutes and working out the best modality for you. Here are the benefits of breathwork (cyclical hyperventilation):

Improved Oxygen Utilisation: The controlled hyperventilation phase is believed to increase oxygen uptake, potentially enhancing the body's ability to utilise oxygen efficiently.

Stress Reduction: The method is often associated with stress reduction and relaxation, possibly due to its influence on the sympathetic nervous system. In a controlled environment, you voluntarily evoke a stress response with the breath hold, which teaches you how to control your stress reaction. This helps you stay calm or reset after something frustrating, or anger-evoking happens throughout your day.

Enhanced Mental Clarity: You can't focus on deep, slow breaths with your monkey brain running wild. You need to focus on each breath because you know you have a 2 or 3 minute breath hold coming up. So if your mind wanders away from the breath, you won't sufficiently oxygenate your body and be able to complete the breath hold. Then, during the breath hold, you must cultivate a clear mind to stay calm and in control, which can lead to increased mental clarity and focus in the hours that follow.

Cognitive (thought) Restructuring

This builds on your mindfulness work. When you say or think, "This is the worst thing ever, why do things always happen to me, etc.? That's where cognitive restructuring comes in. It's about challenging and changing those negative thought patterns.

Everyone faces setbacks, but adopting a victim mentality only reinforces helplessness, doubt, and insecurity. Instead, take a proactive approach. Reframe the situation to see what you can control or learn. Sometimes, a positive outcome may be out of reach, and that's okay. Even then, you can walk away with valuable insights and growth. Remember, every failure is a stepping stone toward becoming stronger, wiser, and more resilient.

Physical Activity and Exercise

When you engage in physical activity, your brain and body release a powerful cocktail of beneficial chemicals. Endorphins function as natural painkillers and mood enhancers, helping to alleviate discomfort and lift your spirits. Dopamine is key in motivation, reward, and pleasure, driving you to pursue goals and relish achievements. Serotonin helps stabilise your mood and fosters a sense of well-being, promoting emotional balance and calm. A simple walk outside can transform your day, offering immediate and lasting stress-relief benefits.

Journaling

Regular expressive writing is a therapeutic outlet, helping you process and navigate pent-up emotions. This practice not only reduces stress levels but also fosters emotional well-being by enhancing self-awareness and emotional resilience. You gain clarity and a deeper understanding of your emotions by putting your thoughts and feelings onto paper.

If you're unsure where to start, incorporating gratitude into your journaling can be a game-changer. Gratitude helps train your brain to notice and appreciate the small things in life, and this shift in focus can profoundly transform how you experience life. Being grateful for what we have can increase happiness, well-being, and life satisfaction while decreasing anxiety, depression, and anger.

To begin a gratitude practice, take a few minutes each day to write down three things you're grateful for. These can be anything from a supportive conversation with a friend to a beautiful sunset. The key is consistency. By acknowledging the good in your life, you can retrain your mind to focus on positivity and appreciation, enhancing your overall mental and emotional well-being.

Having A Goal or Something To Aim At

Aimlessness breeds uncertainty, and uncertainty is the breeding ground for anxiety. The primary cause of anxiety is not knowing what is going to happen in the future or having too many things to deal with at once. Getting clear on your priorities and focusing on what you can change will provide a sense of purpose and direction.

Having a clear aim won't magically make life easy, but it gives your struggles a purpose. It's like turning on the headlights in the dark - you can see where you're going, even if the path is challenging.

Time Management and Task Prioritisation

Effective time management and task prioritisation can significantly enhance productivity and reduce stress. By focusing on high-impact tasks and organising your schedule, you accomplish more in less time and avoid being overwhelmed by last-minute pressures. This structured approach boosts your efficiency and helps you maintain control and balance, leading to a more manageable and fulfilling day.

Eliminate Distractions

Eliminating distractions is a powerful step in managing daily stress because distractions pull us away from tasks, increase mental clutter, and can make even simple tasks feel overwhelming. Constantly shifting focus or responding to interruptions fragments our attention, heightens stress levels, and leads to a sense of unfinished business.

By actively removing distractions, silencing notifications, creating a focused workspace, or setting boundaries, we reduce the "noise" that drains our mental energy. This clears the way for us to work more effectively, stay grounded, and complete tasks more easily, significantly reducing daily stress and fostering a sense of calm and control.

Healthy Lifestyle Choices

Eating a balanced diet will give your body the right fuel to ensure that your brain and body perform optimally without dips in energy and focus. Don't forget that quality sleep is the unsung hero of stress management. It's our nighttime therapy session when we process and deal with the day's events. Neglect your sleep, exercise and nutrition, and you will be a grumpy, unfocused, irrational mess.

Social Support and Connection

Humans are inherently social creatures, and having a strong support network can act as a powerful buffer against the negative effects of stress. Reaching out, sharing your thoughts, and connecting with others eases the emotional burden, helping to melt stress away.

Social support is not just comforting - it's essential. When your emotional health is good, staying motivated to eat well, being productive, and exercising becomes easier. But when you're feeling isolated or emotionally drained, even the best intentions can fall by the wayside. So, never underestimate the power of connection in your stress-management toolkit.

Even though you may be meditating and exercising to reduce the effects of stress, you will still face stressful situations throughout your day.

To reduce or eliminate these feelings of anxiety, anger or overwhelm, there are some simple behavioural tools you can use in the moment to get back in control and face the situation with a clear mind.

Instant Stress Busters To Get In Control Of The Situation

Implementing one or more of the above stress management tools, e.g., meditation, breathwork, or journaling, will undoubtedly help to improve your emotional and mental well-being, but this is usually done in a comfortable and safe space.

But what happens when shit hits the fan, and you find yourself in a situation where you are angry, overwhelmed, irritated, losing or stressed to the eyeballs. This is where you need a couple of tactics or tools that can be implemented at that moment to stay in control of your emotions and focus on what needs to be done.

The best-known strategy for changing one's mental state is to leverage the body's power and ability to positively affect how we feel. Engaging in simple activities like breathing or moving will directly influence your mindset. Don't try to change a negative emotional state with thoughts alone; this takes monk-like conditioning.

You need to use your body to change how you feel, because it is very hard to outthink negative thoughts.

When your flight or fight response is on red alert, and you are in a heightened emotional state, it is hard to turn that off with thoughts alone; for some people, it is impossible. That is why you need to have a couple of well-rehearsed practices that engage the body and breath to calm the nervous system and allow you to get focused and back in charge of your mental state.

When stressed or stuck in our head ruminating, we generally start to take shallow breaths, which leads to a build-up of carbon dioxide and a lack of oxygen. We have very acute receptors that sense this change in the blood, which can signal the release of adrenaline and cortisol in an attempt to move you into action. So all it takes is a few focused deep breaths, and you can quickly reverse those feelings of stress or being overwhelmed and get your head back in the game.

Here is a set of techniques to help refocus your attention and start performing your best again.

The Physiological Sigh: A double inhale, followed by a long, slow exhale.

How to Use: Take a deep breath through the nose, then immediately top it up with a second short inhale. Fully expand the chest and lungs and hold for one second. Finish with a slow, controlled exhale out through the mouth. This fully inflates your lungs, boosts oxygen levels, and allows you to blow off the build-up of CO_2 that increases feelings of agitation.

This simple technique allows you to refocus and regain control of the situation. It is the quickest and easiest to implement and is my go-to method for releasing frustration or anger and refocusing.

Box Breathing (4-4-4-4): This technique focuses on equalising the duration of inhalation, breath retention, exhalation, and the pause between breaths, promoting balance and relaxation.

How to Use: Inhale through your nose for a count of 4. Hold your breath for a count of 4. Exhale completely and steadily for a count of 4. Pause and hold your breath for a count of 4 before starting the cycle again.

Tense and Release Muscles: This technique involves systematically tensing and then releasing muscle groups to reduce physical tension and promote relaxation. I like to combine each contraction with an inhale and exhale.

How to Use: Begin with your toes, tensing the muscles for a few seconds. Release the tension and notice the sensation of relaxation. Move upward, tensing and releasing each muscle group (calves, thighs, abs, arms, etc.) until you stop blowing steam out of your ears and start to relax.

Emotional Freedom Tapping: This relatively new method has proven effective in many trials in calming down people experiencing high-stress symptoms. Although it is not as straightforward as breathing techniques, it can still introduce a sense of calm.

Tap on each acupressure point while focusing on your breath. As you tap on each point - starting with the side of your hand and moving through the 8 points - repeat calming words like "breathe" or "focus." Please refer to page 31 for pressure points and further instructions. This one takes some practice, so work through the sequence a few times and stick at it.

Seeking Professional Help: Remember, it's okay to ask for help. If stress starts to feel like a heavy backpack that you can't take off, professionals are there to help. They can provide personalised strategies and therapies to help you navigate stress more effectively.

Understanding the effects of both acute and chronic stress is crucial for maintaining our overall health and performance. Acute stress can be beneficial, providing the necessary drive to overcome immediate challenges, but chronic stress can significantly damage our physical and mental health.

Unfortunately, in our Western culture and education system, there is little emphasis on using stress-beating strategies, such as meditation, breath work, journaling, and exercise, which are essential for building long-term resilience. Hence, it is up to you to discover the methods that work for you and find a tribe that aligns with your beliefs.

Having stress-buster tools like the physiological sigh and tapping at your disposal equips you to handle high-pressure situations effectively. By practising and integrating these tools into your routine, you can transform stress from a foe into a friend, harnessing its energy when needed and mitigating its harmful effects when it becomes overwhelming.

Give yourself time to meditate... to disconnect, because when you invest in yourself, you invest in your future.
~Dr. Joe Dispenza

Stress Less Challenge -
Improve Your Focus and Stress Levels.

Level 1: Mindful Breathing or Meditation - Dedicate 10-20 minutes each morning to breath work, meditation or journaling practice.

Learn to be present and cultivate a sense of calm and purpose to start the day. This is crucial to ensure you start your day feeling centred and ready to face whatever comes your way.

Create a list of things you want to accomplish, a to-do list, rewrite goals, or set intentions. Whatever provides the most clarity and direction for your day. Pick one and do it for a week!

Level 1.2: Focus on your circle of influence - start identifying where you are wasting mental bandwidth and energy on things that you have no control over and put that time and energy into things you can influence, e.g. training, nutrition, family.

Level 2: Digital Detox - Take a break from electronic devices for at least one hour daily. Disconnect from screens and engage in a non-digital activity. This will create space for mental relaxation and reduce the impact of digital stimuli on stress.

Level 2.1: Nature Connection - Spend that digital detox time outdoors. Do some gardening, go for a walk, or ride. Whether it's at the beach, in the park, or on a nature walk, immerse yourself in the natural environment. Harness the therapeutic benefits of nature to alleviate stress and enhance well-being.

Level 3: Gratitude Practice - End your day by jotting down three things you're grateful for and three things you did well that day. Reflect on the positive aspects of your day. Foster a mindset of gratitude, shifting focus from stressors to positive experiences.

Pillar 3 - Nutrition And Hydration

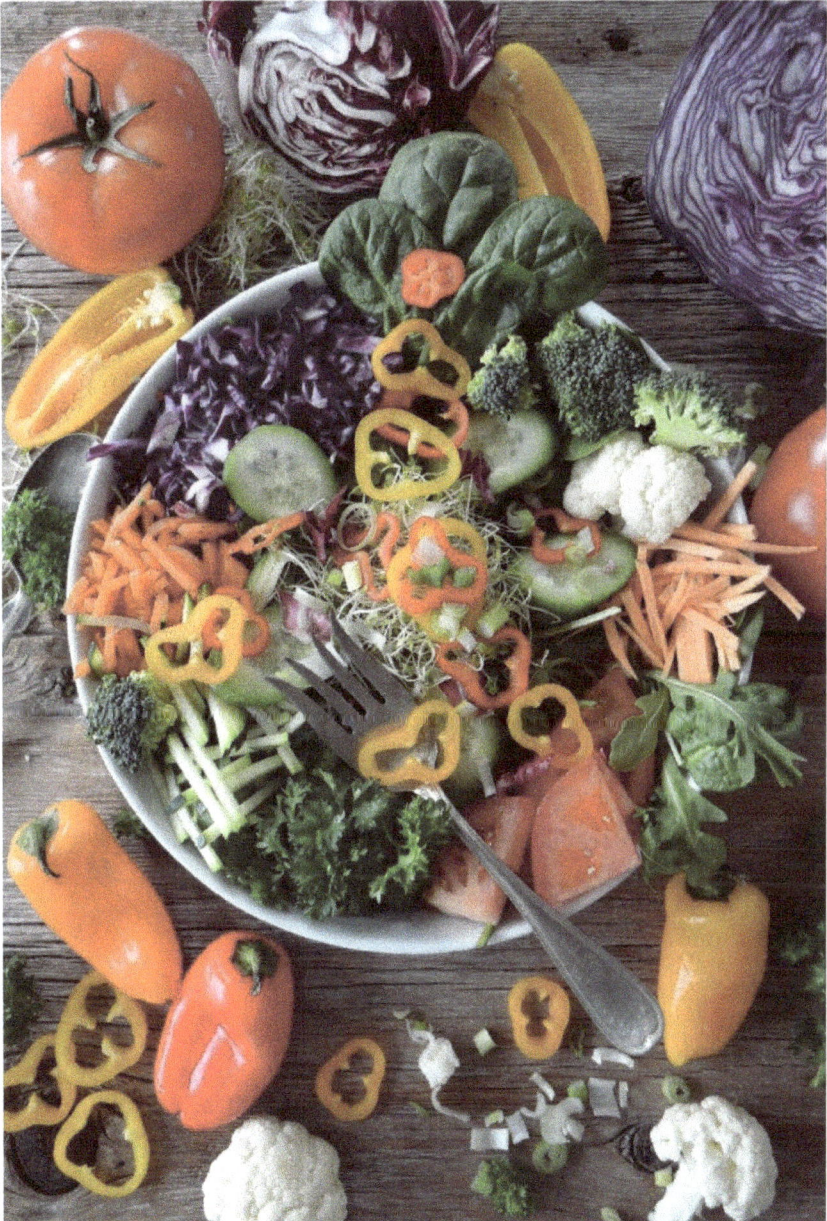

Part 1 - Eat Whole Foods, Mostly Plants, And Don't Overconsume.

In the not-so-distant past, our ancestors had to hunt, gather, and work for their sustenance. Food was a precious and often hard-earned resource. But today, we find ourselves in a world where food is abundant, calorie-dense and cheap, and there lies the problem.

Our modern food industry has perfected the science of creating highly refined, hyper-palatable food-like products. Over the past 50 years, the emphasis has shifted from quality to quantity, prioritising shelf stability and irresistible flavours engineered to override natural satiety signals and keep us coming back for more.

The result is an overabundance of processed, convenience-focused foods that flood our takeaway restaurants and supermarkets but lack the essential nutrients our bodies truly need. It's a paradox where people are overfed yet undernourished, and it's high time we open our eyes to this reality. In this pillar, we'll delve into the journey from our ancestors' struggle for sustenance to our modern dilemma of abundance without true nourishment.

It's a bit like a plot twist in a Hollywood movie. Our once beneficial sustenance has morphed into a villain, silently chipping away at our health. But fear not! We can change the script. The key to our well-being lies in the mantra, "Eat whole or minimally processed foods, mostly plants, and don't overconsume." It's time to swap those processed villains for natural, wholesome superheroes.

Busting The Fast Food Myth

Picture a typical scene at McDonald's: teenagers laughing and joking, all while munching on the iconic Big Mac. But are these meals enough to fuel our bodies? No. The truth is that many of us have become disconnected from the true source of our food and its purpose - to nourish our bodies and minds. It's time to re-educate ourselves about nutrition and the power of whole foods.

The Western Diet: A Tale Of Unhealthy Choices

Imagine a scale. On one side, we have processed foods, added sugar, and unhealthy fats; on the other, we have colourful fruits, vegetables, whole grains, nuts, and seeds. Shockingly, the Western diet has tipped this scale heavily towards the former, leading to an unfortunate plot involving obesity, heart disease, and diabetes. But we can rebalance this scale and rewrite our health story. Plus, we can ensure we are fuelling our bodies to perform at their best.

Protein: The Hero In Our Food Story

Protein is like the lead character in our body's action movie. It's crucial for repairing and building muscle, but just like in a movie, the quality of the lead character matters. Here's a list of common foods and their approximate protein content:

Food Type (100 grams)	Grams of Protein
Chicken breast (cooked, skinless)	31 grams
Chicken thigh (cooked, skin off)	25 grams
Beef (lean cuts, cooked)	26 grams
Lean beef mince (cooked)	21 grams
Pork chop (cooked)	24 grams
Salmon (cooked)	25 grams
Tuna (in oil, drained)	24 grams
Lentils (cooked)	9 grams
Quinoa (cooked)	4 grams
Chickpeas (cooked)	8 grams
Tofu	8 grams
Greek yoghurt	10 grams
Eggs	13 grams
Cottage cheese	11 grams
Almonds	21 grams
Peanut butter	25 grams
Black beans (cooked)	8 grams
250ml milk (full cream)	8 grams

How Much Protein Do You Need and Protein Bioavailability

Imagine you're at a party. Yes, it is a weird and wonderful party full of proteins. Everyone's having a great time, but not all proteins are created equal. Some are the life of the party - they're fully absorbed by your body and put to good use. Others, well, they're shy wallflowers, not fully utilised. This is what we call protein bioavailability.

Now, what determines whether a protein is the life of the party or a wallflower? Well, it depends on the protein source, how it's processed, and who it parties with (other nutrients). Animal-based proteins like whey protein, eggs, and meat are like extroverts. Thanks to their complete amino acid profiles and efficient digestion, they are highly bioavailable.

Plant-based proteins, however, are like introverts. They have lower bioavailability due to digestibility variations and can lack all the essential amino acids.

Plant proteins are contained within the fibrous structure of plant cell walls, making them less accessible to digestive enzymes. This structural complexity, combined with plant fibres and certain anti-nutrients, can reduce the efficiency of protein extraction and digestion compared to animal proteins. Consequently, the bioavailability of plant proteins is generally lower, but with the right preparation, e.g., cooking, soaking, or sprouting, can help improve protein accessibility and absorption.

But hey, even introverts can shine by teaming up with others. Combining different plant proteins can enhance their overall amino acid profile and, if paired correctly, make them more bioavailable.

Complete Versus Incomplete Protein

Have you ever wondered why proteins are labelled as complete or incomplete? Complete proteins contain all nine essential amino acids, the building blocks for cells your body can't create alone. In contrast, incomplete proteins lack one or more of the essential amino acids.

These nine amino acids are essential for maintaining muscle tissue. Without a steady supply, your body might break down precious muscle tissue to meet its needs. Complete proteins mostly come from animal sources, such as eggs, chicken, beef, lamb, and pork. Some plants, including quinoa, buckwheat, and soy, also join the complete protein party.

The Journey of Protein: From Plate to Muscle

Ever wonder what happens to the protein in your steak or scrambled eggs after you eat it? It is a fascinating journey that transforms food into the building blocks that repair and rebuild your body. Understanding this process reveals why planning and proper preparation play a vital role in optimising protein absorption and utilisation.

Cooking is essential to maximising protein digestibility and nutrient absorption. Heat denatures (unfolds) proteins, making them more accessible to digestive enzymes and increasing the availability of amino acids.

The Digestive Adventure

After chewing and swallowing your protein-rich meal, it quickly enters your stomach. Here, powerful stomach acids and enzymes (like pepsin) get to work, breaking the protein into smaller chains of amino acids called peptides. This is the "preparation phase," where raw protein is transformed into more usable forms.

Next, these peptides enter the small intestine, where specialised enzymes continue breaking them down into individual amino acids. These amino acids are absorbed through the intestinal wall and enter the bloodstream. From there, they're whisked away to the liver, the central processing hub that determines how and where they'll be used.

Muscle Repair: The Role of Leucine

One standout amino acid, leucine, plays a central role in muscle repair and growth. Once enough leucine (about 3 grams) is circulating in your bloodstream, it acts as a green light for muscle protein synthesis (MPS), the process of repairing and rebuilding muscle fibres after exercise or daily wear and tear.

This is why consuming sufficient protein at each meal is critical. Without enough high-quality protein, the body may lack the raw materials to stimulate MPS and maintain or grow muscle mass.

Beyond Muscles

Amino acids don't stop at building muscles. They are required to form enzymes that catalyse chemical reactions, hormones that regulate processes like metabolism, and even the components that maintain cellular health and immune function. Every part of your body, from your hair to your heart, relies on amino acids for optimal performance.

Protein Requirements

Well, that's like asking how much fuel a car needs. It depends on the car and the distance you want to cover. Similarly, protein requirements vary based on age, sex, and activity level. Protein requirements should be presented in a range, not one singular number, as consuming within a range of grams is more realistic and achievable. Consuming 20g under or over the calculated range is acceptable, considering there are small amounts of protein in many food items. Here are the recommended grams per day based on activity levels.

Sedentary Adults: Imagine you're a couch potato, just sitting around all day. You'd need about 0.8 grams of protein per kilogram of body weight daily. This is the recommended baseline requirement to survive.

Recreational Exercisers: If you hit the gym or run a few times per week, you'd need between 0.8 and 1.2 grams of protein per kilogram of body weight per day. I recommend a minimum of 1 gram kg/bw. It's like filling up your tank; you need more than normal to cover extra distance.

Endurance Athletes: For endurance athletes engaging in long-distance running or cycling, your body needs more protein for muscle repair and recovery. So, you'd require 1.2 - 1.6 grams of protein per kilogram of body weight daily. This could go to 1.6 - 2 g/kg when the training volume is high and competition phases.

Resistance Trainers: If you are trying to increase your muscle mass with strength and resistance training four or more times a week, you need more protein to facilitate growth and repair. In this case, you'd need 1.6 - 2 grams of protein per kilogram of body weight daily.

Team sports: When you train both on the field and in the gym, you are asking a lot of your body, and it will require large amounts of protein (and carbs) to recover from all the stressors it experiences in a week.

After reviewing further studies on protein intake and performance, it appears that the ideal protein intake for active individuals to maximise performance, control appetite, and increase lean muscle mass is **2 - 2.4 grams** of protein per kilogram of body weight per day.

Optimal Daily Protein Intake For Muscle Gain

It's important to understand that a daily protein intake of 3 g/kg isn't likely to help you build more muscle than a daily protein intake of 2.2 g/kg.

To support muscle recovery and growth, it is recommended that protein be consumed within two hours after resistance training. Elevated protein needs can persist for up to 24–48 hours post-workout, making it essential to distribute protein intake evenly across meals throughout the day for optimal recovery and results.

However, if you are trying to lose weight, you will need to be in an energy (calorie) deficit, so having a higher protein intake will help minimise the lean muscle mass loss that will come with cutting weight.

Embrace Good Fats for a Healthier You!

Fats are the unsung heroes in the journey towards optimal health and peak performance. Far from being dietary foes, these powerhouse nutrients are vital to our existence. They serve as the body's energy reserves, guardians of our brain power, builders of our hormones and allies in the fight against inflammation. This next section unveils the fascinating world of fats and how they are indispensable to our physical vitality and mental health.

Healthy Hero Fats

Polyunsaturated Fats: These are the superstars of heart-healthy fats. They're found in salmon, mackerel, flaxseeds, walnuts, and chia seeds. These fats contain essential omega-3 and omega-6 fatty acids that are great for brain health, reducing inflammation, and supporting cardiovascular function.

Monounsaturated Fats: These fats are a secret weapon for overall well-being. Found in foods like avocados, olive oil, almonds, and peanuts, they're known for improving cholesterol balance by lowering LDL (low-density lipoprotein) and potentially raising HDL (high-density lipoproteins). These fats support heart health and may even aid in weight management.

Saturated Fats: While these should be consumed in moderation, they're not all bad. Coconut oil, for instance, contains saturated fats that are different from those in animal products. Other sources include lean cuts of meat, dairy, and dark chocolate. These can be part of a balanced diet but should be limited to maintain heart health.

The Bad Fats

Unhealthy Trans-unsaturated Fats: Let's call them the villains of the fat world - causing harm wherever they go. The primary source of trans fats is processed foods made with partially hydrogenated oils. These harmful fats are created by adding hydrogen to vegetable oils, transforming them into a more solid form. Companies favour trans fats because they extend the shelf life of processed foods, are cheap to produce, can be reused in fryers, and enhance flavour and texture in some products. Foods that contain trans-fat to eat less of:

- Deep-fried foods
- Biscuits, cakes and pastries
- Takeaway foods, such as hamburgers, pizza, deep-fried chicken and hot chips.
- Foods that list hydrogenated oils or partially hydrogenated vegetable oils.

Now that you know the cast of characters, it's all about making smart choices. Embrace those healthy fats to fuel your high-performance journey while keeping trans fats at arm's length. Including enough healthy fats in your diet is important for all the following reasons.

Hormone Production: Healthy fats are also vital for hormone production. They are necessary for synthesising steroid hormones like estrogen, testosterone, and cortisol. These hormones regulate various bodily functions, including metabolism, immune response, and reproductive health. Cholesterol is the support act for all these hormones, so I want to share the following to demonstrate how important it is.

Cholesterol is often misunderstood, but it's a vital lipid (fat) that plays a key role in many of the body's essential functions. As a crucial component of cell membranes, cholesterol is necessary for synthesising hormones like estrogen, testosterone, and cortisol. It also contributes to producing vitamin D and bile acids, which aid digestion.

As cholesterol is a lipid and hydrophobic (meaning it does not dissolve in water), it requires a protein carrier to travel through the bloodstream. These protein carriers, known as lipoproteins (LDL and HDL), allow cholesterol to be transported effectively within the water-based environment of blood. These lipoproteins transport cholesterol around the body, but an imbalance can lead to health risks. Remarkably, around 80% of the cholesterol in your body is produced by the liver and intestines, with only about 20% coming from your diet. This highlights how essential cholesterol is for maintaining hormonal balance, digestive health, and overall well-being.

Brain Health: Polyunsaturated fats, particularly omega-3 fatty acids, are your brain's best friends. They help maintain the structure of brain cell membranes, ensuring smooth communication between brain cells. This, in turn, supports cognitive function, memory, and overall mental well-being.

Heart Health: Healthy fats play a crucial role in supporting cardiovascular health. They help reduce the risk of heart disease by lowering LDL cholesterol levels, reducing triglycerides, and increasing

HDL cholesterol. These effects contribute to improved blood lipid profiles, reduced arterial inflammation, and overall better heart function.

Anti-Inflammatory Powers: Inflammation is a major player in many chronic diseases. Polyunsaturated fats, especially omega-3s, are renowned for their anti-inflammatory properties. They can help ease conditions like arthritis and even reduce the risk of inflammatory disorders.

Cell Builders: Did you know that fats make up a significant part of the outside layer of most cells in your body? They're the guardians of your cells, maintaining their structure and function.

Vitamin Absorption: Fats are needed to absorb fat-soluble vitamins A, D, E, and K. They ensure that we get the most out of our food.

Skin Health: Fats help maintain skin elasticity and hydration, reducing dryness and inflammation.

Energy Levels: Fats provide a concentrated energy source, which is especially important for long-term endurance and overall vitality.

Here is a broader list of foods to include in your diet that have been shown to improve all the health benefits listed above.

- **Avocados**
- **Eggs** (especially the yolk)
- **Fatty Fish**
- **Olive Oil**
- **Chia Seeds**
- **Flax Seeds**
- **Coconut Oil**
- **Dark Chocolate**
- **Nuts**
- **Pumpkin Seeds**
- **Sesame Seeds**
- **Tahini** (sesame seed paste)
- **Ghee** (clarified butter)
- **Full Fat Yoghurt**

Carbohydrates: The Energy Powerhouse

Carbohydrates are like the supercharged car our hero rides in an action-packed chase scene. They fuel our bodies, providing the energy we need to take on the world. But remember, not all carbs are created equal. Whole grains, fruits, and vegetables are your best bet. On the other hand, refined grains and added sugars are like the speed bumps that slow down our hero, so it's best to avoid them.

In a balanced diet, carbohydrates should come from whole, unprocessed sources like fruits, vegetables, whole grains, and legumes, which provide essential nutrients, fibre, and sustained energy without the unhealthy downsides.

Like every captivating movie plot, our food story has good and bad actors. So, revel in your favourite treats occasionally, but ensure most of your carbs come from fruits, vegetables, and whole grains. This way, you can treat yourself and not feel like you are missing out and being punished.

The Power of Carbohydrates: Fuelling Your Body Wisely!

Carbohydrates are the body's preferred energy source, but remember, not all carbs are your friend. Here are my favourite carbohydrates to consume and which ones I avoid.

Eating whole grain products: When grains are refined, they don't retain the bran (husk) and germ, which are rich in fibre, vitamins, minerals, and antioxidants. These components contribute to better digestion, more stable blood sugar levels, heart health, and overall nutritional intake. Opting for whole-grain varieties can provide significant health benefits when choosing bread, pasta, or cereals.

Vibrant Veggies: Filling your plate with colourful vegetables is like adding a rainbow of nutrients to your diet. Think of carrots, broccoli, sweet potatoes, and pumpkin as your nutritional bodyguards, providing essential vitamins, minerals, and fibre you and your gut need.

Fruit Frenzy: Enjoy nature's candy all year round. There are so many delicious fruits available that change with each season. Fruits offer natural sugars, fibre and a host of micronutrients and antioxidants, making them perfect energy-boosting sidekicks.

Side note: if you can eat the skin, don't cut it off!

Legume Power: Beans, lentils, and chickpeas are unsung nutrition heroes. They are packed with fibre, complex carbs, and plant-based protein and are a great way to boost your protein intake, especially if you are not eating animal products.

Snack Smart: Choose smart snacks like fruit, carrot sticks, or a handful of your favourite nuts. They're satisfying, nutrient-packed sidekicks for hunger pangs.

Carbohydrates To Avoid

White Bread: In white flour production, the wheat kernel is stripped of its bran (outer layer) and germ (nutrient-rich core), leaving only the starchy endosperm. This refining process removes most of the fibre, healthy fats, vitamins, and minerals.

Pastries and Baked Goods: Think of doughnuts, muffins, croissants, and many commercially baked goods. The combination of sugar, fats and salt results in a calorie-dense, nutrient and fibre devoid food.

Sugary Cereals: Many breakfast cereals, especially those marketed to children, are high in sugars, have no fibre and lack essential nutrients. It's the same as having dessert for breakfast.

Processed Snack Foods: Lollies, chips, crackers, and snack bars are often high in unhealthy fats, sugars, and refined carbohydrates. Check labels for added sugars and unhealthy fats.

Soda or Sugary Drinks: These are a significant source of refined sugars and empty calories. Regular consumption leads to weight gain and diabetes.

Fruit Drinks or Juices: While fruit juices may seem healthy, many are high in added sugars and lack the fibre in whole fruits. Avoid fruit juices that have had the fibre or pulp removed.

Fast Food: Burgers, fries, and many other fast-food options are often packed with unhealthy carbs and fats, deep-fried, and have high salt content. The underlying problem is they are super palatable, calorie-dense, and don't contain any fibre, so you eat more than you need without realising it.

The foods we eat profoundly influence how we look, feel, and perform. If you're facing any health issues, it's crucial to examine your diet and its effects on your gut health because that is where most problems originate. I'll share a story of how changing my diet changed my life.

One of the most impactful decisions I've made came when I was just 13 years old. Like many teenage boys, I started experiencing acne, and after trying various face washes and creams with little success, we turned to our family doctor for advice. His simple yet powerful recommendation was to spend 10-15 minutes in the sun each day and avoid processed foods with added sugar.

I followed his advice, cutting out soft drinks, lollies, junk food, and sugary cereals while my mom packed my lunches with nutritious options like sandwiches, fruit, nuts, muesli bars and dried apricots. Removing all the unhealthy processed foods helped clear up my skin but, more importantly, improved my energy and focus and set the foundation for lifelong healthy eating habits and a healthy gut.

I ate a diverse range of vegetables and fruit and spent a lot of time outside. Which, unbeknown at the time, led to a healthy gut. It also means I have an excellent immune system, and I'm proud to say I haven't been to a GP for a cold or flu in more than 20 years and have not taken antibiotics since I had my wisdom teeth out when I was 19. If you're facing issues with your health or energy levels, start by examining your diet and how it's affecting your gut health.

The Quiet Achiever: Dietary Fibre

Dietary fibre is the indigestible part of plant foods and has many health-promoting benefits. It is filling yet has no calories. It absorbs and retains water, aiding satiety. It slows the emptying of the stomach, decreasing hunger without adding calories.

It resists absorption in the small intestine before undergoing complete or partial fermentation in the large intestine. The bacteria in the large intestine, collectively known as the gut microbiome, need this to feed on and, as we now know, play a crucial role in promoting mental and physical health. Here are some ways these bacteria, which need fibre to thrive, contribute to your health and performance.

1. Nutrient Synthesis: The gut microbiome is involved in synthesising (producing) specific vitamins and nutrients, such as B vitamins and vitamin K. These compounds are essential for various physiological functions, including energy metabolism and blood clotting.

2. Digestion and Nutrient Absorption: Gut bacteria assist in breaking down complex carbohydrates and fibres that our digestive system cannot do on its own. This process releases short-chain fatty acids (SCFAs), which provide an energy source for the cells lining the large intestine to keep your gut working effectively. SCFAs have anti-inflammatory and neuroprotective effects, potentially benefiting both mental and physical health.

3. Immune System Support: Most of the immune system resides in the gut, where gut bacteria are crucial in regulating immune responses. These beneficial microbes help train immune cells to recognise and appropriately react to pathogens while distinguishing between harmful invaders and benign substances.

This balance is essential for preventing unnecessary inflammation, reducing the risk of autoimmune reactions, and maintaining overall health. A healthy gut supports a strong, resilient immune system, which impacts everything from digestion to mental well-being.

4. Neurotransmitter Production: The gut-brain axis communicates between the gut and the central nervous system. Gut bacteria produce neurotransmitters such as serotonin and GABA, which play a key role in regulating mental well-being and helping you get to sleep and stay asleep.

5. Metabolism and Weight Regulation: Certain gut bacteria have been linked to increased or decreased metabolism and body weight regulation. A diet high in sugar and low in fibre creates dysbiosis of the gut microbiome, which can speed up the onset of obesity.

6. Inflammation Regulation: A balanced gut microbiome helps regulate inflammation in the body. Chronic inflammation is associated with various health issues, including mental health conditions such as depression and anxiety.

7. Stress Response: The gut microbiome can influence the body's response to stress. Research suggests that a healthy balance of gut bacteria may contribute to resilience against the negative effects of stress.

8. Protection Against Pathogens: Gut bacteria play a protective role by preventing the colonisation of harmful pathogens. They compete for resources and produce substances that inhibit the growth of potentially harmful microorganisms.

In summary, fibre is fundamental for a balanced gut microbiome, which in turn impacts immune health, mental wellness, weight management, and protection against pathogens, underscoring its crucial role in overall health.

The British and American Gut Project studied the diets of thousands of people, assessing how different dietary patterns were associated with different health outcomes. One of the most interesting findings was around fibre. The recommended fibre intake for an adult is 30-35g a day, but the study showed that the amount of fibre is not as important as the variety.

Different plants have different fibres, so eating more plants will automatically diversify the types of fibre you eat. The study showed that people who ate the largest variety of plant foods were found to have the healthiest microbiomes and were likely to report the best health outcomes. It suggested that aiming for 30 different plant-based foods a week is optimal for fibre diversity.

Fibre Content In Common Foods

Food Type	Average Serving Size	Amount of Fibre Per Serve
Sweet Potato	1 medium (150g)	4g
Pumpkin	1 cup diced	2.7g
Carrots	1 medium (60g)	2.3g
Broccoli	1 cup chopped	5.1g
Green Beans	1 cup cooked	3.4g
Peas	1 cup	8.8g
Corn	1 medium cob (80g)	2.7g
Lettuce	1 cup shredded	0.5g
Silver Beet	1 cup chopped	3.4g
Strawberries	1 cup	3.3g
Apples	1 medium (182g)	4.4g
Oranges	1 medium (131g)	3.1g
Peach	1 medium (150g)	2.3g
Pineapple	1 cup of chunks	2.3g
Brown Rice	1 cup cooked	3.5g
White Rice	1 cup cooked	0.6g
Wholemeal bread	1 slice	1.9g
White bread	1 slice	0.3g
Avocado	1 medium (200g)	13.5g
Oats	1 cup cooked	4g
Lentils	1 cup cooked	15.6g
Chickpeas	1 cup cooked	12.5g
Spaghetti Pasta	1 cup cooked	2.5g
Mixed Nuts	100g	9g

How To Make The Right Choices

Riding The Wave (aka Urge Surfing) is a powerful concept for managing cravings, particularly when trying a new diet, cutting out junk food, or reducing calories to lose weight. This approach involves acknowledging the craving, understanding its temporary nature, and learning how to navigate it without giving in.

The urge could be to gamble, shop, watch porn, drink beer or the desire to eat (usually junk food), which we will focus on here. The urge to eat can sometimes be overwhelming, especially when tired or stressed, even when there's no hint of physical hunger.

Cravings often feel overwhelming, like a mighty wave crashing over you, and even though it might not feel like it at the time, you have the power to choose whether you act on the urge or not. Of course, to make this decision, you need first to notice that you're having a craving. Then, once you've acknowledged it, you ask yourself a series of questions - If I act on this craving, is this in alignment with the sort of person I want to be? Will it take me closer to my goals?

The key is to learn that cravings are temporary - they will pass if you don't act on them. Here are the steps to ride the wave.

Recognise the Craving: The first step is to realise that you're experiencing a craving. This awareness is crucial because it allows you to pause before reacting. Recognise it as a natural response instead of trying to suppress or ignore the craving. Focusing on where the craving is experienced (where there is increased arousal). For example, with food, it may be the mouth (salivating), the stomach (due to hormone release) and the brain (due to the anticipation of receiving a reward).

Acknowledge: Once you recognise the craving, acknowledge and observe the feeling the particular craving experience brings. Notice how it feels in your body and mind. Do you feel restless, tired, stressed, bored? By becoming an observer of your craving, you create a mental distance between you and the urge. Focus on where you feel the craving physically.

Is it a tightness in your chest? A sensation in your stomach? By pinpointing the physical sensations, you reduce the emotional power of the craving.

Ride the Wave: As the craving peaks, remind yourself that it will pass. Imagine it as a wave that rises and then falls. You don't need to fight the wave; you must ride it until it subsides. The more you practice this, the better you become at managing cravings. Use deep breathing techniques or mindfulness exercises during the peak of the craving. For example, inhale deeply for a count of four, hold for four, and exhale for four. This gets you focused on something else, calms your nervous system and helps you ride out the wave.

This is also a great time to ask yourself whether giving into the craving will be voting for the person you want to be. So ask yourself, "What small step can I take right now that will take me closer to the person that I want to be?"

Refocus Your Attention: After acknowledging and riding the wave, redirect your attention to something else. Engage in an activity that absorbs focus and removes your mind from the craving. This could be anything from going for a walk to calling a friend or working on a task that requires concentration. Having a list of go-to activities when a craving strikes is a great idea.

Reflect and Learn: After the craving has passed, reflect on the experience. What triggered the craving? How did it feel to ride the wave? Each time you successfully manage a craving, you build confidence in your ability to handle future urges.

Riding the wave is effective because it shifts your mindset from resisting or battling cravings to accepting and navigating through them. This approach reduces the emotional charge of the craving and empowers you to handle urges without relying on willpower alone.

Now that you have a behavioural tool to overcome snacking and binge eating let's look at a practical way to ensure you make good food choices.

Learn To Read and Interpret Food Labels

Remember to be a food detective! Checking food labels for ingredients, macronutrients, and added sugars is a great strategy for fine-tuning what you put in your body and avoiding ultra-processed foods.

Understanding how to interpret food labels is crucial for making informed and health-conscious dietary choices. The nutrition information panel becomes a valuable tool when comparing similar foods, such as breakfast cereals, canned goods, or pre-prepared meals.

Additionally, the ingredient list, presented in descending order of weight, provides insight into the product's composition. Be attentive to added substances, including food additives like colours, flavours, preservatives, and emulsifiers. By carefully examining food labels, you empower yourself to make healthier choices that align with your nutritional needs and dietary preferences.

Don't rely on the Australian Health Star Rating (HSR) to determine your food choices. Despite its widespread use, the system has notable limitations. It only applies to packaged goods, meaning fresh, minimally processed foods are not included.

If your diet revolves around food from packets and boxes and you rely on the stars on the box or packet to inform your food intake, you are eating too many processed foods. If you value your health, don't rely on the stars on the box or packet to guide your nutritional intake. Instead, focus on whole, minimally processed foods for better health outcomes.

How to Use the Label:

- **Step 1**: Start with the ingredients list to identify the main components and hidden unhealthy additives (sugar, salt, food additives, colours, thickeners).

- **Step 2**: Check the per 100g column to evaluate macronutrient ratios. Focus on protein, fibre, and sugar levels to assess overall healthiness.

- **Step 3**: Evaluate energy and portion size to match your nutritional needs.

Red Flags on Labels:

A long list of unrecognisable or chemical-sounding ingredients often means the food is highly processed and lacks nutrients. It has multiple types of sugars or sweeteners listed in different forms. Words like "artificial," "modified," "hydrolysed," or "enriched" often indicate unnecessary additives or nutrient stripping during processing.

If you can't identify or pronounce most of the ingredients, it's a good sign to avoid the product.

Nutrition Information

Total Fat ▶
Generally choose foods with less than 10g per 100g.
For milk, yogurt and icecream, choose less than 2g per 100g.
For cheese, choose less than 15g per 100g.

Saturated Fat ▶
Aim for the lowest, per 100g. Less than 3g per 100g is best.

Other names for ingredients high in saturated fat: Animal fat/oil, beef fat, butter, chocolate, milk solids, coconut, coconut oil/milk/cream, copha, cream, ghee, dripping, lard, suet, palm oil, sour cream, vegetable shortening.

Fibre ▶
Not all labels include fibre. Choose breads and cereals with 3g or more per serve

Servings per package – 16
Serving size – 30g (2/3 cup)

	Per serve	Per 100g
Energy	432kJ	1441kJ
Protein	2.8g	9.3g
Fat		
Total	0.4g	1.2g
Saturated	0.1g	0.3g
Carbohydrate		
Total	18.9g	62.9g
Sugars	3.5g	11.8g
Fibre	6.4g	21.2g
Sodium	65mg	215mg

Ingredients: Cereals (76%) (wheat, oatbran, barley), psyllium husk (11%), sugar, rice, malt extract, honey, salt, vitamins.

Ingredients ▲
Listed from greatest to smallest by weight. Use this to check the first three ingredients for items high in saturated fat, sodium (salt) or added sugar.

◀ 100g Column and Serving Size
If comparing nutrients in similar food products use the per 100g column. If calculating how much of a nutrient, or how many kilojoules you will actually eat, use the per serve column. But check whether your portion size is the same as the serve size.

Energy
Check how many kJ per serve to decide how much is a serve of a 'discretionary' food, which has 600kJ per serve.

Sugars
Avoiding sugar completely is not necessary, but try to avoid larger amounts of added sugars. If sugar content per 100g is more than 15g, check that sugar (or alternative names for added ◀ sugar) is not listed high on the ingredient list.

Other names for added sugar: Dextrose, fructose, glucose, golden syrup, honey, maple syrup, sucrose, malt, maltose, lactose, brown sugar, caster sugar, maple syrup, raw sugar, sucrose.

◀ Sodium (Salt)
Choose lower sodium options among similar foods. Food with less than 400mg per 100g are good, and less than 120mg per 100g is best

Other names for high salt ingredients: Baking powder, celery salt, garlic salt, meat/yeast extract, monosodium glutamate, (MSG), onion salt, rock salt, sea salt, sodium, sodium ascorbate, sodium bicarbonate, sodium nitrate/nitrite, stock cubes, vegetable salt.

Image courtesy of - www.eatforhealth.gov.au

The table below provides the macronutrient ranges that should make up the standard diet recommended by the Australian Government.

Macronutrient	Recommendation (Estimated Energy Requirements)
Protein	15 - 25% of total EER
Carbohydrates	45 - 65% of total EER
Fat	20 - 35% of total EER

The next table provides alternative ranges for macronutrient recommendations based on varying research, allowing a more tailored approach. The macronutrient ratios can be manipulated to suit your preferences and goals and subsequently improve adherence.

Macronutrient	Expanded Recommendation (Estimated Energy Requirements)
Protein	15 - 35% of total EER
Carbohydrates	20 - 60% of total EER
Fat	20 - 55% of total EER

I want you to understand the importance of learning about nutrition to ensure you are correctly fuelling your body. Refrain from settling for a generic meal plan from a trainer or friend at the gym or the internet. Your need for proteins, fat, and carbohydrates will depend on your goals and preferences and can change based on your stage of life.

I want to show you that your diet's macronutrient ratio will depend on your goals. So, let's compare the macronutrient breakdown of three other diet examples to the Australian Dietary Guidelines recommendations.

AUSTRALIAN DIETARY GUIDELINES

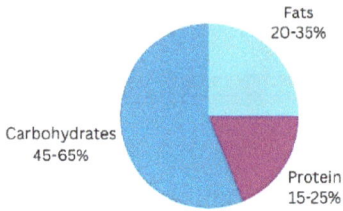

MUSCLE GAIN

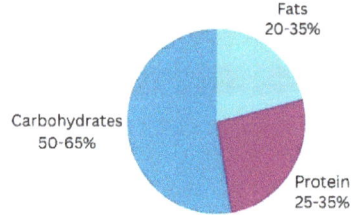

WEIGHT LOSS

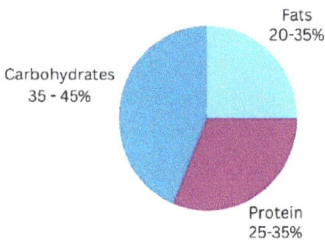

KETO

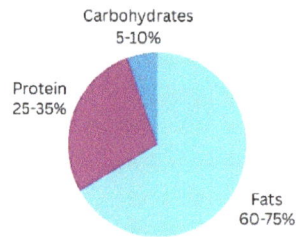

Proteins, fats and carbohydrates contain a specific amount of energy per gram when broken down during digestion. Fat is more energy-dense than protein and carbohydrates. The following table shows how much energy, represented in kilojoules and calories, is found in each macronutrient per gram. Alcohol is considered a macronutrient because it releases energy when broken down. This is the definition of empty calories, as alcohol has zero nutritional benefits.

Regarding nutrition and exercise, kilocalories (kcal) and calories equal the same amount of energy. You may also express energy as kilojoules (kJ), with one calorie or kcal equalling 4.18 kJ.

Energy Source (Per Gram)	Calories (Cal)	Kilojoules (KJ)
Carbohydrate	4	16.72
Protein	4	16.72
Fat	9	37.62
Alcohol	7	29.26

How Much Should You Be Eating?

Now that you have an overview of the three macronutrients and how to use them to make up your daily intake, you need to work out how much energy (food) you need to eat to be at your best and hit your goals. Fuel your body like a high-performance machine, and it can run at full throttle and not break down.

Two calculations determine how much fuel you need: the Basal or Resting Metabolic Rate (BMR) and the Estimated Energy Requirement (EER).

We'll use the Harris-Benedict equation to estimate your daily energy needs (EER) in kilojoules, aiming to provide a useful benchmark. While consuming close to this target is ideal, hitting the exact number daily isn't essential. Unless you're preparing for a specific goal, like stepping on stage for a bodybuilding competition, don't let calorie counting overshadow the importance of eating a clean, mostly unprocessed diet. Prioritise nutrient-dense, whole foods over obsessing about exact numbers - this approach will better support long-term health and performance.

BMR, often interchangeably used with Resting Metabolic Rate (RMR), is the baseline energy expenditure at complete rest. It's the energy your body expends for essential functions like maintaining body temperature, circulating blood, and breathing, all without any cognitive input. Now, EER takes centre stage as the total energy required, encompassing BMR, the thermic effect of digesting food, and energy spent on physical activity. It is a number tailored for active people.

Step 1: Calculating the BMR

There are different equations to determine the BMR for men and women, based on the assumption that men have a higher percentage of lean body weight than women (which increases BMR in men).

Men	BMR = 278 + (57.5 x W) + (20.93 x H) - (28.35 x A) kJ/day.
Women	BMR = 2741 + (40 x W) + (7.74 x H) - (19.56 x A) kJ/day.

W = Weight in kilograms (kg), H = Height in centimetres (cm), A = Age

STEP 2: The second step is multiplying the BMR by the physical activity level (PAL) to establish the final EER. Use the table below to multiply the individual's BMR with their corresponding PAL.

Estimated Energy Requirements = BMR x PAL

Physical Activity Level (PAL)		Description	Example of Occupation
Very Sedentary	1.4-1.5	Exclusively sedentary activity/seated work with little or no strenuous leisure activity.	Office employees
Light Active	1.6-1.7	Sedentary activity/seated work with occasional walking and standing but little to no strenuous activity.	Uni Student, Office worker, driver
Moderate Activity	1.8-1.9	Predominantly standing and walking	Waiter, tradesman, teacher/coach, and nurse.
Heavy to Vigorous Activity	2.0-2.4	Significantly active with additional strenuous exercise	Your occupation plus additional strenuous exercises.

If your activity level for work/occupation fits into levels 1.4 – 1.9 and you exercise strenuously (30-60 mins, 4-5 times a week), change your selection to the next highest activity level. For example, James is a waiter with a PAL of 1.8, but he goes to the gym four times a week for 45 minutes. This means he would fall into the next highest category of heavy activity, with a PAL of 2.0. If a client does not participate in regular exercise, they will stay at the level according to their occupation.

Case Study: Ben

A 22-year-old male who is 178cm tall and weighs 76kg attends lectures and studies during the day, trains hard at football practice twice a week, and hits the gym four times a week, plus a game on the weekend. His goal is to get to 80kg.

Step 1: BMR = 278 + (57.5 x W) + (20.93 x H) - (28.35 x A)

BMR = 278 (57.5 x 76) + (20.93 x 178) - (28.35 x 22)

BMR= 278 + 4370 + 3726 - 623.7

BMR = 7750 kj/day

Step 2: EER = BMR x PAL

EER = 7750 x 1.9 (1.7 + strenuous exercise)

EER = 14 725 kj/day or 3522 calories/day.

Finally, suppose you want to lose or gain approximately 500g of weight per week. In that case, it is recommended that 2,000kJ needs to be subtracted (weight loss) or added (weight gain) to your calculated Estimated Energy Requirements. You are better off starting with a smaller reduction in energy than big changes for weight loss. It is easier to adapt to and still gives you room to reduce energy intake. This avoids going into a huge deficit, where you can plateau, slow your metabolism and feel empty and tired.

Step 3: Adjust for Weight Goals

Since Ben's goal is to gain weight (target 80 kg), let's add 2000 kJ (approximately 500 calories) per day to his **EER** to aim for a weekly gain of 500 g.

Adjusted EER = 14,725 + 2000 = 16,725 kJ/day or 4000 calories/day.

Additional Guidance

- **Gradual Adjustments**: Starting with smaller increments for weight gain, like adding 500-1000 kJ (120-240 calories) initially, is often easier to adapt to and may prevent excess fat gain. This way, Ben can monitor his progress and adjust intake as needed.

- **Nutrient-Dense Foods**: Since Ben is working to gain lean mass, prioritise nutrient-dense foods high in protein, healthy fats, and complex carbs to support his training.

Now that you know your daily energy intake requirement, it's time to identify the ratio of macronutrients that make up your diet. The first step is determining how much protein you need to meet your daily requirements. Once you establish how much protein you need, you can calculate how many calories or kilojoules this will total. Then, based on your goals or preferences, split the remaining energy required between carbs and fats based on your preferences.

Daily Protein Requirement = weight x activity level or body composition goal

= 80kg x 2.2 = 176 g/d

= 176g x 16.72 kj = 2943 kj/day

Hence, if your EER is 14 725 kj/day, your protein portion is 2943 kj.

2943 / 14725 = 0.2 x 100 = 20% protein

Protein intake is 20% of total macronutrients. Based on your goals, you can decide on the proportion of carbohydrates and fats you need in your diet. With this knowledge, you can fine-tune your nutrition plans to fuel performance, optimise recovery, and support body composition goals.

Calculating BMR and EER may sound a little complex, but fear not, there are tools to help with the process of calculating and tracking the food you require. Many people tend to have a relatively consistent diet, often cycling through the same 20-30 foods over two weeks.

Hence, tracking your food intake for a short period, like one or two weeks, can provide valuable insights into your eating habits. It can help you identify patterns, understand portion sizes, and make informed decisions about your nutrition.

So, while long-term tracking isn't necessary for everyone, a brief monitoring period can be highly beneficial in understanding and improving your diet.

Food is the most impactful lever to pull when it comes to managing or maintaining weight. Exercise is undeniably valuable for overall health, fitness, and longevity, but nutrition takes the lead in directly influencing weight. Focusing on food quality, caloric intake, and meal timing is essential for weight loss, maintenance, or gain. If I were to quantify the impact of nutrition versus exercise on changing body composition, it would be 70/30 in favour of diet.

While exercise can enhance health and metabolic efficiency, our food choices ultimately dictate the results we see on the scale. A consistent exercise routine will support overall wellness, but emphasising a strategic approach to nutrition will deliver the most significant and sustainable results.

To help track and manage what you are eating, here are the best-rated calorie counter apps by verywellfit.com

Best Calorie Counter Apps of 2024

- Best With Lots of Features: My Fitness Pal
- Best for Healthy Eating Support: Lifesum
- Best for Diet Support: My Net Diary
- Best for Weight Loss: Lose It!
- Best for Simplicity: Control My Weight
- Best Completely Free: Calorie Counter by Fat Secret

Now that you know about the three macronutrients - protein, fat, and carbohydrates - there is another category of nutrients called micronutrients.

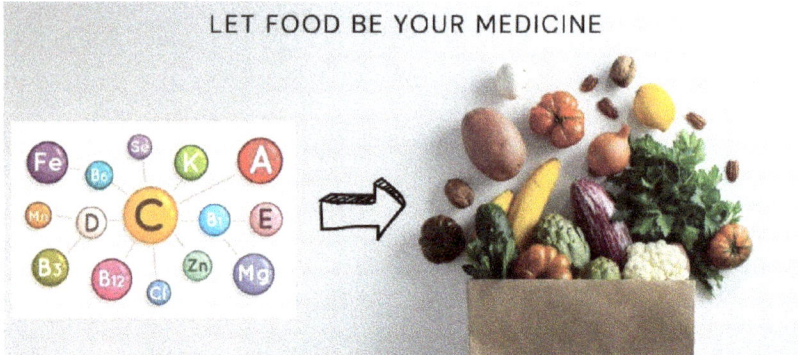

LET FOOD BE YOUR MEDICINE

Micronutrients

Micronutrients are essential nutrients that our bodies need in relatively small amounts but play a colossal role in maintaining good health. The body requires both vitamins and minerals to function correctly. The difference is that vitamins are organic compounds made by plants and animals. Minerals are inorganic compounds that originate from the earth and are obtained from water and soil. Minerals make their way into our diet through plants that absorb them from the soil. When we eat these plants directly or consume animals that have fed on them, we take in these essential nutrients through our food.

There are 13 different vitamins, which can be categorised into two different groups:

1. Fat-soluble vitamins:

- Vitamin A (also known as retinol)
- Vitamin D (also known as cholecalciferol)
- Vitamin E (also known as tocopherols)
- Vitamin K.

2. Water-soluble vitamins:

- Vitamin B1 (also known as thiamine)
- Vitamin B2 (also known as riboflavin)
- Vitamin B3 (also known as niacin)
- Vitamin B5 (also known as pantothenic acid)
- Vitamin B6 (also known as pyridoxine)
- Vitamin B9 (also known as folate/folic acid)
- Vitamin B12 (also known as cyanocobalamin)
- Biotin
- Vitamin C (also known as ascorbic acid).

There are fundamental differences between fat-soluble and water-soluble vitamins. Fat-soluble vitamins refer to vitamins that require dietary fat for their absorption. They are absorbed alongside dietary fats, and excess is stored in the body's fatty tissue. Excess consumption can lead to toxicity because fat-soluble vitamins are stored in the body. It is, therefore, important to consume fat-soluble vitamins in small amounts and frequently rather than in large quantities sporadically.

Water-soluble vitamins dissolve in water, meaning they require water for absorption and transportation. Hence, if there is too much water-soluble vitamin, it will be excreted out of the body when you pee. As a result, we need to consume water-soluble vitamins daily to avoid deficiency. Nature knows best when it comes to providing the body with nutrients. This is why you need a wide variety of whole foods to get all the necessary vitamins and minerals.

Why Vitamins Are Important

Vitamin A: Supports vision, immune function, and skin health. It is found in carrots, sweet potatoes, and spinach.

B Vitamins (B complex): Vital for energy production, metabolism, and a healthy nervous system. Sources include whole grains, eggs, and leafy greens.

Vitamin C: Boosts the immune system, aids collagen production, and acts as an antioxidant. Citrus fruits, strawberries, and capsicum (bell peppers) are excellent sources.

Vitamin D: Crucial for bone health and immune function. The only foods that contain substantial amounts of vitamin D are oily fish, eggs, and UV-light-exposed mushrooms, e.g., field mushrooms.

Vitamin E: Acts as an antioxidant, supporting skin health and protecting cells. Nuts, seeds, and spinach are rich sources.

Vitamin K: Essential for blood clotting and bone health. Common sources are leafy greens, broccoli, and soybeans.

Why Minerals Are Important

Essential minerals are micronutrients that the human body requires in small amounts regularly. There are two major categories of essential minerals: trace and major minerals. Trace minerals are necessary for the human body in smaller amounts than major minerals, although both play fundamental roles in maintaining health.

Major Minerals	Trace Minerals
• Sodium	• Iron Manganese
• Calcium	• Fluoride
• Chloride	• Chromium
• Potassium	• Molybdenum
• Phosphorous	• Zinc
• Magnesium	• Iodine
• Sulphur.	• Selenium
	• Copper

Sodium: A vital electrolyte that plays an essential role in enzyme operations and muscle contractions. It is required to maintain a healthy fluid balance in the body. Common sources are table salt, anchovies, olives, feta cheese, bread, stock cubes, and canned fish.

Potassium: Another important electrolyte that works alongside sodium to maintain healthy blood pressure and fluid balance in the body. It also aids the transmission of electrical pulses for proper nerve and muscle function. It is found in cocoa, dried fruit, nuts and seeds, legumes, dairy, potatoes, avocados, and bananas.

Magnesium: A significant cofactor in more than 300 biochemical reactions, including protein synthesis, muscle and nerve function, blood glucose control, and blood pressure regulation. It is required for energy production and muscle contraction/relaxation. Magnesium is found in various food sources, including green leafy vegetables, legumes, nuts, fish, avocados and bananas. Research shows that one in three people do not consume enough magnesium for their body's needs, so pay particular attention to this one.

Calcium: Vital for bone health, muscle function, and nerve transmission. It is found in dairy, green leafy vegetables, broccoli, tahini and almonds.

Iron: forms an essential component of haemoglobin, the protein in red blood cells responsible for transporting oxygen throughout the body. It's especially abundant in meat, poultry, and seafood, which provide heme iron, a form the body absorbs efficiently. Iron is also present in plant foods such as whole grains, nuts, seeds, and leafy green vegetables, but these sources contain non-heme iron, which is less readily absorbed.

Consuming plant-based iron with vitamin C-rich foods, like citrus fruits, berries, or capsicum, can enhance absorption. Maintaining adequate iron levels is critical for energy production, immune function, and cognitive health. It is particularly important for individuals with higher iron needs, such as menstruating women, athletes, and those on plant-based diets.

Zinc: plays vital roles in growth and development, protein synthesis, immune function, and wound healing. It also supports both male and female reproductive health while being essential for the senses of taste and smell. Zinc is crucial for enzyme function and DNA synthesis, making it key to cellular repair and renewal. It's also an antioxidant, helping to reduce oxidative stress, which supports skin health and may have anti-inflammatory effects. Zinc-rich foods include oysters, red meat, poultry, legumes, mushrooms, and fish. Since the body doesn't store zinc, regular intake through diet is essential, particularly for individuals at higher risk of deficiency, such as vegetarians, pregnant women, and those with digestive conditions.

Selenium: Selenium acts as a powerful antioxidant, helping to protect cells from oxidative damage and supporting immune system function. It's also essential for thyroid health, as it plays a role in producing thyroid hormones that regulate metabolism. Selenium is involved in DNA synthesis and may contribute to reducing inflammation in the body. Great sources of selenium include Brazil nuts (which are exceptionally rich in selenium), seafood, whole grains, eggs, and poultry.

What Happens When You Are Overnourished With All The Wrong Foods?

Being overweight is mainly caused by an energy imbalance. This is when too much energy is taken in through food and drink, and not enough energy is expended through exercising and your basal metabolic rate. Factors that contribute to excess weight gain and obesity can be attributed to rapid weight gain during childhood, lack of nutritional education, poor sleep, hormonal imbalances, having parents who are overweight or obese, and exposure to the marketing of unhealthy foods.

A growing body of evidence highlights that easy access to highly palatable and calorie-dense food and drink is a big issue. So, to avoid being another health statistic, ensure you are well informed, make the best choice of the available food, and avoid highly processed foods. If you neglect to be aware of the food you put in your body, you are limiting your mental and physical capabilities.

Don't Be Fooled By The Marketing

The tactics of today's food industry bear a striking resemblance to those once employed by the tobacco industry. Just as cigarettes were marketed as glamorous and cool, big food corporations have used similar strategies to promote processed foods as desirable, nutritious, and even essential.

Let's take a step back in time. In the 1980s, as the health risks of smoking became undeniable, major tobacco companies began diversifying into the food industry. Philip Morris acquired Kraft and General Foods, while R.J. Reynolds purchased Nabisco. These acquisitions didn't just expand their empires - they brought the tobacco industry's expertise in marketing and addiction engineering into the food sector.

What followed was the deliberate development of highly processed, hyper-palatable foods designed to drive repeat consumption, paired with misleading labels, celebrity endorsements, and vibrant packaging to create the illusion of health and necessity.

Fast forward to today, and ultra-processed foods have become the new battleground for public health, much like tobacco was decades ago. While individuals are encouraged to make healthier choices, the reality is that the food environment is flooded with options engineered to be addictive and nutritionally hollow. Processed foods are marketed as convenient and tasty solutions for modern life, but the reality is they are prioritising corporate profits at the expense of public health.

It's crucial to understand that these companies' primary goal is profit - not your well-being. Strategic marketing, food engineering, and consumer demand have combined to normalise the consumption of unhealthy, addictive foods. Every dollar spent on fast food or highly processed products contributes to the wealth of these corporations while potentially compromising your health.

The lesson is clear: the food industry thrives on keeping consumers uninformed and hooked. Achieving optimal health requires us to see through the marketing, make informed decisions, and prioritise whole, nourishing foods over convenience and corporate interests. Empower yourself by choosing foods that truly fuel your body and support your long-term health.

Finding The Right Diet In The Age Of Abundance

For the vast majority of human evolution, food scarcity was the norm. Our biology is hardwired to seek and store energy, a survival mechanism that ensures we can endure periods of famine. Yet, in the modern environment of endless food availability, an unprecedented change occurring in just the last 0.01% of our evolutionary timeline, we now face a different challenge: managing abundance. This requires a conscious and intentional approach to nutrition, often involving some form of sacrifice or restriction.

To maintain or lose weight in this environment, you must make deliberate choices about what to restrict. While the specifics of the restriction can vary, the ultimate goal is the same: create a diet that allows you to be vibrant and healthy and not get fat. Whether you choose to:

Restrict Calories Directly: Tracking your intake to ensure you eat less than you burn.

Restrict Timing: Limiting eating windows through approaches like intermittent fasting and time-restricted eating.

Restrict Specific Foods or Macronutrients: Avoid certain foods, e.g., pasta, milk chocolate, soft drinks(soda), or restrict whole macros such as carbohydrates, fats, or alcohol.

The key point is this: there is no perfect diet. Each approach has its pros and cons, and the best diet for you is the one that aligns with your lifestyle, preferences, and goals while being sustainable in the long term. For example, low-carb diets often stand out as particularly effective for weight loss and appetite control, but they are not universally suited to everyone.

The takeaway is that some form of restriction is inevitable in today's food-abundant world. However, the restriction doesn't have to feel punishing. By choosing an approach that resonates with your values and habits, you can build a sustainable nutritional strategy that supports your health and performance goals and fits seamlessly into your life.

5 Key Principles To Guide Your Food Choices

1. **Balanced Nutrition:** Aim to include at least 30 different plant-based foods in your diet each week. These include fruits, vegetables, whole grains, legumes, nuts, herbs, and spices. Variety ensures a broad range of nutrients and fibre types, which support a diverse and robust microbiome.

2. **Eat Whole, Unprocessed Foods Most Of The Time:** Whole foods are your best friends. They're like the purest form of nutrition. Fruits, veggies, whole grains, and lean proteins are loaded with the good stuff your body needs without the additives and preservatives that overly processed foods have.

3. **Portion Control:** Pay attention to portion sizes. It's like managing the fuel your body needs. Even healthy foods can lead to weight gain if you eat them excessively.

4. **Mindful Eating:** Practice mindful eating to enhance your relationship with food. It's not just about what you eat, but also how you eat. Savour each bite, eat slowly and be attentive to your body's signals of hunger and fullness. Share meals with family and friends, and relish how delicious healthy food can be.

5. **Eats Lots of Fibre:** Fibre promotes regularity by aiding in the movement of food through your digestive system, preventing constipation. Additionally, fibre acts as a prebiotic, nourishing beneficial gut bacteria and contributing to a healthy microbiome. It also helps promote satiety, reduce calorie intake, and support weight management.

Adherence Is The Holy Grail

Numerous studies have shown that adherence is the most critical factor in any diet's success. It's not about adhering to a specific set of dietary rules but finding a lifestyle approach that resonates with you. Whether it's the flexibility of intermittent fasting, the plant-powered vitality of a vegetarian diet, or the metabolic benefits of a low-carb approach, the key is choosing a dietary pattern you can commit to long-term.

Rather than chasing short-term fixes, aim for long-term solutions that support lasting mental and physical health. Food should be enjoyed and shared with friends and family, not cause isolation due to rigid dietary rules. There will be times when you can't eat exactly as you usually do, stay flexible and make the best choice from what's available.

The Power Of Experimentation

Finding your ideal dietary approach may require some experimentation. It's an opportunity to explore various foods and meal timing while listening to your body and observing how it responds. Pay attention to your energy levels, digestion, and overall feelings of satiety. Remember, it's a journey, and what works for you today may evolve as your body's needs change over time.

Seek Guidance and Support

Seeking guidance from healthcare professionals, such as dietitians or nutritionists, can be immensely valuable. They can help you navigate the vast sea of dietary information, provide personalised recommendations, and ensure that your chosen approach aligns with your health and performance goals.

In the quest for the perfect diet, let go of the notion that if a particular approach doesn't work for you, you are somehow flawed. Often, it's simply a matter of miscalculation. You might think you're eating 2000 calories but are actually consuming more or less. We are notoriously poor judges of our total intake, so don't throw in the towel if a month goes by and results are slow to appear. Like exercise, a healthy diet requires consistent review, evaluation, and adjustment.

On this journey of self-improvement, experiment with different approaches, but beware of those who claim their diet is the perfect solution for everyone. When someone insists their diet is the answer, it often reveals a shallow understanding of nutrition. Avoid falling into the trap of following an influencer's "amazing" diet simply because it worked for them. Instead, focus on finding what works for you.

Remember, a sustainable diet is not a 12-week challenge - it's a lifelong commitment to thriving. By embracing a diet rich in whole, unprocessed foods and maintaining a well-balanced nutritional approach, you build a foundation for resilience, vitality, and health. Each meal is more than satisfying a craving; it is an investment in your future, fostering energy, protecting against disease, and enhancing your quality of life for years to come.

Here's to making choices that empower and enrich our bodies, one nutritious bite at a time!

Part 2 - Supplements: Supporting Your Mental And Physical Performance

In the pursuit of optimal health and well-being, many people turn to dietary supplements to fill nutritional gaps and boost both mental and physical performance. While supplements can indeed play a valuable role in supporting specific health goals, it's crucial to understand when and why to use them effectively.

Remember, supplements are not a replacement for a varied and balanced diet. They should not be a fallback for poor dietary habits, a lack of food variety, or reliance on highly processed foods lacking essential nutrients. Instead, supplements should be viewed as complementary tools to reinforce a foundation of nutritious eating and healthy lifestyle choices.

Since I could afford them, I've used supplements to support my training and performance. Through experience, I learned that while some supplements can enhance health and performance, others offer minimal or no benefits. Working in a health and sports supplement store for three years allowed me to refine my understanding of what works, when to use it, and which products are backed by evidence.

Thanks to extensive research and reliable findings from countless studies and human trials, we now have a more accurate, evidence-based approach to recommending and using supplements. This clinical data guides my recommendations, allowing me to suggest supplements with proven efficacy for performance and recovery confidently.

My supplement stack varies throughout the year, but my weekly staples are protein powder, creatine monohydrate, fish oil, zinc, magnesium, and a stress adapt product. I also use a pre-workout consisting of cognitive and blood flow enhancers when needed.

There are many supplements on the market, and most don't make the following list. I focus on single ingredients and effective dosage amounts rather than blended pre-made products, so you know what to look for when buying yours. When buying pre-made supplements, please read the label to see the main ingredients and their dosage amounts. The key ingredients are often underdosed, containing too many fillers, binders, artificial colours and sweeteners. So, after reading the following pages, you will know how much of those key ingredients are needed to be effective and when is the best time to use them.

It is important to do your own research and find out what you are putting in your body. This is easy to do these days with some reliable sources of information on supplements, such as www.examine.com.

Let's dive into the details of each supplement, highlighting their benefits and recommended dosages for optimal outcomes.

Creatine Monohydrate

Creatine primarily boosts energy metabolism by helping to quickly regenerate ATP, the body's main energy currency for high-intensity exercise. ATP (adenosine triphosphate) is the molecule that delivers energy within cells. When ATP is used for energy, it loses a phosphate group and is converted into ADP (adenosine diphosphate) or AMP (adenosine monophosphate). Creatine, stored in cells as phosphocreatine, steps in to help replenish ATP. It does this by donating a high-energy phosphate group to ADP, converting it back into ATP and allowing for sustained energy during intense activities.

By increasing the pool of cellular phosphocreatine, creatine supplementation accelerates the recycling of ADP into ATP, quickly replenishing cellular energy stores. This increased energy availability can lead to improvements in strength and power output. Increasing the available muscle stores of phosphocreatine causes faster regeneration of ATP, allowing for decreased rest time between activities and increased energy for repeated bouts of exercise.

The benefits of creatine extend beyond skeletal muscle, affecting nearly all body systems, including the central nervous system, which comprises the brain and spinal cord. The evidence suggests that creatine intake may improve performance on memory and cognitive tasks.

Dosage: Two standard methods of supplementation can increase creatine storage in the body. There is no need to cycle on and off creatine.

1. In the loading phase, 20 - 25 grams of creatine (0.3 g/kg day) (every 4 hours) are consumed for 5-7 days, followed by 3-5g per day as a maintenance dose.

2. Start with the maintenance dose of 3 - 5g daily and continue for as long as required. Reaching creatine muscle saturation will happen more slowly, and total muscle saturation can take as long as 4 weeks.

Timing: Some evidence demonstrates taking a 5g dose 1–2 hours before training will improve strength output. However, you will still benefit from taking 5g each day regardless of the time you consume it.

Common questions and misconceptions about creatine supplementation: what does the scientific evidence really show?

https://jissn.biomedcentral.com/articles/10.1186/s12970-021-00412-w

Beta-Alanine

Beta-alanine supplementation offers multiple performance benefits, particularly for high-intensity exercise lasting 1–10 minutes. By boosting muscle carnosine levels, beta-alanine enhances endurance and delays fatigue by buffering the buildup of hydrogen ions that accumulate during intense activity.

This buffering helps stabilise muscle pH, reduce acidity, and allow athletes to maintain performance and push harder for longer. This is especially beneficial for activities like 400–1500 meter running and 100–400 meter swimming, where prolonged power output is key.

Since beta-alanine is the limiting factor for carnosine synthesis, supplementing with it effectively raises carnosine levels in the body.

Timing and Dose: Studies have found a range of 3.2–6.4 grams per day of beta-alanine to be effective for enhancing exercise performance. To optimise carnosine stores, a loading dose of 4–6 grams per day divided into doses of 2 grams or less for a minimum of 2 weeks is suggested.

To avoid paraesthesia (the tingles), 0.8–1.6 grams of beta-alanine every 3–4 hours is recommended. The longer you use beta-alanine, the less you will feel the tingles. Sustained-release formulations are also available that permit greater doses without the risk of paraesthesia. Although beta-alanine is commonly included in pre-workout supplements, the timing of ingestion does not influence its effectiveness. It appears that having it alongside carbohydrates and protein enhances muscle carnosine levels.

Blood Flow Enhancers

This is a category of nitric oxide boosters that can be beneficial in optimising athletic performance. Enhanced nitric oxide production results in vasodilation, the widening of vessels, improving blood flow and oxygen delivery. Enhanced blood flow can improve exercise performance and endurance by supplying muscles with more oxygen and nutrients. Improved circulation can aid in removing metabolic waste products, potentially enhancing recovery after intense physical activity.

Athletes frequently turn to nitric oxide enhancers like citrulline, arginine, and betaine, among a few others, to harness these physiological advantages and achieve peak performance during aerobic and anaerobic activities.

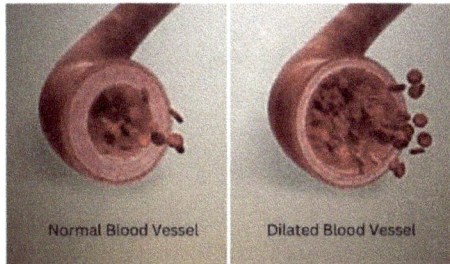

Normal Blood Vessel   Dilated Blood Vessel

Arginine: When you take arginine as a supplement, it is absorbed in the small intestine and then processed by the liver. During this process, the liver can metabolise a significant portion of the arginine, reducing the amount that reaches circulation. This means less arginine is available for conversion to nitric oxide.

Citrulline: Citrulline is not subjected to significant metabolism by the liver. It is readily absorbed in the intestines and directly enters the bloodstream. Once in the bloodstream, citrulline is taken up by the kidneys, where it is efficiently converted to arginine. Citrulline supplementation results in a more sustained increase in plasma arginine levels than direct arginine supplementation. This leads to a more consistent and effective enhancement of nitric oxide production.

The ironic upshot is that citrulline is a better booster of blood arginine levels than arginine. Plus, it comes without arginine's side effects, which can include fairly intense digestive distress for some people.

L-Citrulline or Citrulline Malate: L-citrulline is often combined with malate, an intermediary of the Krebs cycle. Supplementing with malate could theoretically support ATP production, potentiating L-citrulline's benefits. It is unclear whether citrulline malate is superior to citrulline as there is currently no research directly comparing the two.

Timing and Dosage: Based on current research, a recommended dose is 3–6 grams per day of L-citrulline or approximately 8 grams per day of citrulline malate. The dose varies depending on the form because 1.75 grams of citrulline malate provides 1 gram of L-citrulline. The remaining 0.75 grams are malate.

Protein Powders - Whey, Collagen, and Plant

Consuming protein powder post-workout enhances recovery and lean muscle mass gains, especially for those regularly engaging in resistance training. These powders offer a concentrated protein source, which delivers enough leucine to activate muscle protein synthesis and aids individuals in achieving their daily protein goals. In the context of low-carbohydrate diets, protein powders become invaluable. They enable individuals to boost protein intake without compromising carbohydrate limits, which is crucial for muscle preservation and overall health on low-carb diets.

Another noteworthy benefit is their role in appetite control and weight management. Protein's satiating effect helps regulate appetite and reduce overall caloric intake. Therefore, protein powders effectively support weight management goals, offering a convenient and versatile solution for individuals striving to optimise their nutritional intake.

Whey Protein is a high-quality, well-absorbed source of protein that's very useful for hitting targeted daily protein goals. Due to its complete amino acid profile and quick absorption, whey protein is generally considered the most effective in aiding muscle repair and growth. Whey Protein Isolate is refined to contain less lactose and is easy to digest.

Collagen Protein can support the repair of muscle tissue but is particularly beneficial for strengthening and repairing surrounding connective tissues, including joints, tendons, ligaments, and skin. It provides key amino acids, like glycine and proline, that are essential for synthesising collagen fibres, enhancing the durability and elasticity of connective tissues. Collagen is also easy to digest and supports gut health, making it ideal for those with digestive sensitivities. Additionally, as a non-dairy protein source, it's a great option for individuals who are lactose or dairy intolerant.

Plant-based proteins include Soy, Pea, Rice, Hemp, and many combination blends. The blended powders generally contain all the essential amino acids, are less granular than in years past and are nicer to consume. Companies are now using alternative protein sources, such as pumpkin and watermelon seeds, resulting in some great products.

Plant proteins can be a suitable option for those with specific dietary preferences, but careful selection and combination of plant protein sources may be required to ensure a complete protein. Ultimately, the best choice depends on individual needs, dietary restrictions, and preferences.

Suggested Dosage: Based on the current evidence, we conclude that to maximise muscle growth (hypertrophy), one should consume protein at a target intake of 0.4 g/kg/meal across a minimum of four meals in order to reach a minimum of 1.6 g/kg/day. Using the upper daily intake of 2.2 g/kg/day spread out over the same four meals would necessitate a maximum of 0.55 g/kg/meal. So, for most people, this would equate to a 20 – 40 gram serving of protein.

The notion that the human body can only digest or utilise 20 grams of protein per meal is a misconception. Research indicates that while the body can absorb and digest larger amounts of protein, the rate of effectiveness of muscle protein synthesis may not proportionally increase with higher single-meal protein intakes.

Carbohydrates

Carbohydrates can be a powerful supplement to enhance athletic performance, particularly in high-intensity or endurance-based activities lasting over 60 minutes. By ingesting carbohydrates, the body's primary fuel source, you can delay fatigue and maintain optimal power output. This is especially critical for prolonged events such as marathons, cycling races, and ultra-endurance activities. The carbohydrate strategy will vary depending on the duration and intensity of the sport.

For most field sports lasting less than 90 minutes, carbohydrate loading or high carbohydrate intake throughout the game is not necessary. As long as athletes are well-fed with a carbohydrate-rich meal 2–3 hours before the game, their glycogen stores will likely be sufficient to sustain performance. During games, consuming 20–30 grams of carbohydrates is sufficient to maintain energy levels. Hydration leading up to and during the game is often more critical than carbohydrate supplementation.

During prolonged activities, the best source of carbs comes from combining glucose and fructose, as this allows for the highest carbohydrate oxidation rates to enhance energy availability and overall performance. The oxidation rate of carbohydrates is 1–1.2 grams per minute, so 60 grams of carbs per hour is sufficient in most situations and hopefully avoids gastrointestinal discomfort.

Timing and Dose:

Duration of Exercise	Amount of Carbohydrate Needed	Recommended Type of Carbohydrate
30-75 minutes	None or small amounts	Hydration is more critical.
1-2 hours	30 grams per hour	Glucose or maltodextrin
2-3 hours	60 g per hour	Maltodextrin or glucose & Fructose in a ratio of 2:1
3 or more hours	90 grams per hour	It is important to have sucrose or maltodextrin & fructose (2:1) to maximise oxidation rates and avoid GI discomfort.

Caffeine

Caffeine triggers impressive physiological responses, including reduced pain perception, sustained attention, increased alertness, and enhanced mood and energy levels. It also stimulates the release of adrenaline, which heightens drive, increases fat oxidation and improves muscle contractility, subsequently increasing strength output.

Suggested Dosage: If you are new to caffeine, start with a dose of less than 100 milligrams. Espresso shots generally contain 60 to 80 milligrams of caffeine.

Based on the research, the optimal dose for sports performance benefits is 3–6 mg per kilogram of body weight (approximately 200–400 mg in a 70 kg person), taken around 60 minutes before exercise. Using a dose at the low end of this range, approximately 3 mg/kg of caffeine before exercise (approximately 200 mg in a 70 kg person), achieves the benefits along with the lowest risk of side effects.

If you are unsure about what supplements you should be using, it is always advisable to consult with a sports nutritionist before incorporating any new supplements into your regimen. They can provide personalised guidance based on your needs, goals, and any underlying health conditions that must be considered.

General Health Supplements To Fill The Gaps In Your Diet.

In addition to sports performance supplements, certain general health supplements play a vital role in supporting vitality, mental well-being, and overall health - especially in addressing nutritional gaps commonly found in modern diets. Here is a list that appears to be needed across the general population.

Fish Oil (Omega-3 Fatty Acids)

Omega-3 fatty acids offer a trifecta of benefits for athletes. Firstly, they possess anti-inflammatory properties, helping to reduce exercise-induced inflammation and expedite recovery. Secondly, they contribute to joint health by reducing stiffness, promoting lubrication, and supporting cartilage integrity. Lastly, crucial for brain health, these fatty acids support cognitive function, focus, and mood, ultimately positively impacting athletic performance.

Suggested Dosage: The recommended dosage of omega-3 fatty acids is around 1-3 grams per day. The dosage range will vary based on your desired outcome and activity levels.

Vitamin D: We spend a lot of time indoors these days and get very little sunlight at certain times of the year, which can result in a deficiency in vitamin D. This is how Seasonal Effective Disorder comes about.

Vitamin D is essential for maintaining healthy bones, supporting the immune system, and regulating mood. The best form of Vitamin D is synthesised after being in the sunshine, but if you live inside or the weather is constantly overcast or rainy, use a supplement.

The ideal daily dose of vitamin D should correspond to its recommended daily allowance (RDA), which is currently 400–800 IU (10–20 micrograms - µg) daily. However, this may be too low for many adults. For moderate supplementation, a standard daily dose of 1,000–2,000 IU (25–50 µg) of vitamin D3 is sufficient to meet most people's needs.

Zinc: An underrated essential mineral that is vital in maintaining optimal health. It supports the immune system, helping defend the body against infections and illnesses while promoting wound healing and tissue repair. Zinc is crucial for proper growth and development, as it is involved in DNA synthesis and cell division. Additionally, zinc contributes to healthy skin, vision, and reproductive health, supporting fertility and hormone regulation. Its antioxidant properties help combat oxidative stress and protect cells from damage.

The recommended daily zinc intake is 8 mg/day for females and 14 mg/day for males. Up to 40 mg/day is generally safe for short-term needs or specific health goals but should be monitored.

Probiotics: Probiotics are beneficial bacteria that live in the gut and support digestive health. Good health starts with a healthy digestive tract. Having the right bacteria in your gut has been linked to improved weight management, immune function, and mood regulation. If you are not supporting the probiotics you take with a fibre-rich diet, you are sending them on a suicide mission.

Prebiotics: Essential non-digestible fibres or compounds that serve as a food source for beneficial bacteria in the gut. They promote the growth and activity of specific strains of bacteria that are beneficial for gut health. In other words, prebiotics act as "fuel" for the existing beneficial bacteria in the gut or the Probiotics you are taking. Prebiotic fibre-rich foods are crucial for feeding and nourishing the beneficial bacteria in your gut. Good sources of prebiotic fibre include onions, garlic, bananas, asparagus, leeks, whole grains, legumes, and flaxseeds.

Magnesium: This is an essential mineral and one of the body's most abundant nutrients, playing a vital role in over 300 enzymatic reactions. It acts as an electrolyte, supporting crucial functions such as energy production (ATP), glucose metabolism, and DNA and protein synthesis. Magnesium is key for muscle and nerve function, bone health, heart health, and overall nervous system regulation. Additionally, it contributes to immune function, blood sugar balance, and even the synthesis and activation of vitamin D. In short, magnesium is a powerhouse mineral, integral to keeping the body's systems balanced and functioning optimally.

Several forms of magnesium supplements are available, and their bioavailability varies, so make sure you use the best source possible. Here are some common forms of magnesium and their potential benefits:

1. Magnesium Citrate is one of the most popular and well-absorbed forms of magnesium.

2. Magnesium Glycinate or di-glycinate is well-absorbed and less likely to cause digestive discomfort than other forms. It is often recommended for individuals seeking to support relaxation and improve sleep quality.

3. Magnesium Malate is involved in energy production, making this form of magnesium potentially beneficial for individuals looking to support muscle function and combat fatigue.

4. Magnesium L-Threonate has been gaining attention for its potential to cross the blood-brain barrier and enhance brain magnesium levels. Some studies suggest that it may improve cognitive function and memory.

5. Magnesium Orotate is often used in cardiovascular health supplements because it can support heart health and improve energy metabolism.

As for dosage, the recommended daily intake for adults can vary depending on age and gender. For adult men, 400-420 mg per day and for women, 300-320 mg per day.

B Vitamins: Enhancing Energy Production and Brain Function

The B-group or B-complex vitamins consist of 8 of the 13 water-soluble essential vitamins. All of these vitamins play crucial roles at the cellular level, including in the production of ATP. These vitamins are also vital for brain function, DNA synthesis, and red blood cell production.

B vitamins are commonly found in multivitamin supplements, which can make it easy to inadvertently consume more than needed if you're taking multiple products. Thankfully, because they are water-soluble, toxicity is rare, as excess amounts are typically excreted in urine. However, it's still important to check the dosages on supplement labels and be mindful of commonly included B vitamins like B6, B12, and folate to avoid unnecessary intake.

Additionally, some individuals may have genetic variations, such as the MTHFR polymorphism, that reduce their ability to methylate B vitamins like folate and B12, making these nutrients less bioavailable. For these individuals, methylated forms of B12 (methylcobalamin) and folate (methylfolate) are better absorbed and utilised by the body. If you suspect this applies to you, DNA tests are available that identify your ability to methylate, detoxify, and much more.

Doubling up on supplements without expert advice can lead to unnecessary intake or imbalances. Speak with a dietitian, naturopath, or pharmacist to ensure you're getting the right types and dosages of vitamins and minerals for your individual needs. Remember, more isn't always better - taking the proper amount is key to safely enjoying the benefits of supplements.

Supplements To Improve Alertness and Memory

A group of supplements called nootropics has shown positive results in improving focus, attention, and memory. They are great to use before a game, training, performance, or even a serious study session. Use the right one at the right time, and you will be surprised at how they help improve your focus and attention.

Alpha-GPC: a powerful nootropic and performance-enhancing supplement that supports cognitive function, memory, and physical performance. As a precursor to choline, it plays a crucial role in enhancing the production of acetylcholine, a neurotransmitter essential for learning, memory, and muscle contraction.

This makes it particularly valuable for athletes seeking to improve their physical output and those looking to boost mental clarity and focus. When taken before training, Alpha-GPC can increase force production, leading to more effective workouts. It has also been shown to boost growth hormone release when combined with exercise, with a daily dose range of 600 - 1000 mg.

L-tyrosine: This amino acid is metabolised to produce neurotransmitters dopamine and noradrenaline. These brain chemicals are like your mood and motivation regulators.

Multiple studies have demonstrated that L-tyrosine can help to prevent declined cognitive function under stressful, cognitively demanding conditions. So, tyrosine can boost your drive and focus when you're feeling unmotivated or in a challenging situation.

L-tyrosine is usually taken in 500–2000 mg doses approximately 30–60 minutes before any bout of cognitive or physical activity.

Lion's Mane: Used in traditional medicine for centuries, particularly in East Asia. This mushroom is rich in bioactive compounds that stimulate the production of nerve growth factor (NGF) in the brain. NGF plays a critical role in regulating the growth, differentiation, and survival of neurons, which are essential for neurogenesis and neuroplasticity. In simpler terms, Lion's Mane helps stimulate the growth of brain cells and strengthens their connections, continuously enhancing your brain's network and cognitive function.

You can take it as a supplement or add it to your diet before a big study session or when you need to stay sharp at work. For optimal benefits, a daily dosage of 500 to 1000 milligrams is typically recommended.

Huperzine A: This natural compound derived from the Chinese club moss plant is known for its potent cognitive benefits. By inhibiting the enzyme acetylcholinesterase, Huperzine A helps increase acetylcholine levels, a neurotransmitter essential for memory, learning, and mental clarity. This enhancement supports memory retention, learning ability, and sustained focus, making it popular among students and professionals. Additionally, Huperzine A has neuroprotective properties, helping to shield neurons from oxidative damage, which may aid in maintaining long-term brain health.

The typical dosage of Huperzine A ranges from 50 to 200 micrograms per day, often taken in one or two doses. Due to its long half-life, it's commonly recommended to cycle Huperzine A. Use it for 2-3 weeks, followed by a 1-week break to prevent tolerance and overstimulation. Although generally safe, some individuals may experience mild side effects like nausea or headaches, especially at higher doses.

Ginkgo Biloba: Commonly used to support brain health and cognitive function. It works primarily by enhancing blood circulation and increasing oxygen delivery to the brain, which helps nourish brain cells and promote mental clarity. Research has shown that Ginkgo may improve memory, cognitive processing, and attention, particularly in older adults. Additionally, it may reduce mental fatigue and improve mood, making it a popular supplement for maintaining cognitive health.

The typical dosage for Ginkgo Biloba is between 120 and 240 mg daily, usually divided into two or three doses. Ginkgo should be taken consistently for best results, as it may take several weeks to build noticeable effects. However, due to its blood-thinning properties, it's not recommended for individuals taking anticoagulants or those with bleeding disorders, as it may increase the risk of bleeding.

Acetyl-L-Carnitine (ALCAR): This derivative of the amino acid L-carnitine effectively crosses the blood-brain barrier, providing several cognitive benefits. It plays a key role in energy production by helping transport fatty acids into mitochondria, which can enhance mental energy, focus, and endurance, particularly during prolonged tasks.

Studies also show that ALCAR has neuroprotective effects, shielding neurons from oxidative stress and supporting mitochondrial health. This makes it beneficial for long-term brain function and possibly slows cognitive decline in aging populations.

Commonly taken at doses of 500 to 2,000 mg per day, ALCAR is generally well-tolerated and effective for enhancing mental clarity, reducing mental fatigue, and supporting overall brain health, making it a versatile choice for cognitive support.

Herbal Supplements

A broad range of herbal supplements known as adaptogens also improve adrenal function, reduce stress, and improve cognitive function. Below is a list of well-established and more recently studied supplements that can support optimal physical and mental health.

Ashwagandha: scientifically known as Withania Somnifera, is a revered traditional medicinal herb with many health benefits. As an adaptogen, it helps the body manage stress more effectively by regulating cortisol levels. Beyond its stress-relief properties, ashwagandha has also been shown to reduce anxiety, improve mood, and enhance overall mental well-being. In addition, a growing body of evidence supports the efficacy of ashwagandha for improving total sleep time and quality.

The most common dosing recommendation is 600 mg daily, typically divided into two doses: one taken with breakfast in the morning and the other in the evening.

Rhodiola Rosea: Its main benefits are associated with its adaptogenic properties, including reduced stress and fatigue and increased mental performance, particularly under stressful conditions. Rhodiola has an extensive track record for efficacy, with medicinal use dating back centuries, when it was used to promote healing, stress relief, and increased sense of well-being.

Doses as low as 50 mg can be effective for daily fatigue prevention. A higher dosage of 280-680 mg is recommended for acute stress and fatigue relief.

Korean Ginseng (Panax Ginseng): Another popular herb renowned for its adaptogenic properties, it is a powerful ally in managing stress and enhancing overall vitality. It has been extensively studied for its ability to improve cognitive function, boost physical performance, and support immune health. Panax ginseng is typically consumed in daily doses ranging from 200 to 400 mg, with the 400 mg dosage showing the most notable cognitive benefits.

I want to finish this section with a final piece of advice regarding supplementation. Avoid the temptation to introduce multiple new supplements all at once. If you add several supplements simultaneously, it becomes challenging to determine which ones are effective and which are not, and if you have side effects, what is causing it. It can take weeks or months to see the benefits of some supplements, so know what you are taking and how long you need to stick with it to see the benefits.

Part 3 - The Essence of Hydration: The Underrated Performance Enhancer

Water, the elixir of life, forms an intimate bond with our existence because, without it, we die. It is a fundamental element that sustains us, supports our physiological functions, and nourishes our bodies in ways that extend far beyond mere hydration.

By the end of this section, you will have a new appreciation for water because of its many benefits for physical and mental performance. My simplest advice to stay hydrated is to carry a water bottle whenever you leave the house.

The human body is predominantly composed of water, with its percentage varying depending on age, gender, and body composition. On average, water makes up approximately 60% of the total body weight in adults. However, this percentage can range from about 45% to 75%, depending on individual characteristics.

Water is vital for numerous physiological processes and crucial to various body parts. Here are those key areas.

Cells: Water is an essential component of cells, comprising a significant portion of their volume. It facilitates biochemical reactions, helps transport nutrients and waste products, and provides the medium for cellular communication.

Blood: Our bodies' blood is predominantly water. It acts as a transportation system, delivering oxygen, nutrients, and hormones to cells while removing waste products for elimination. Adequate hydration is crucial for maintaining optimal blood volume and circulation.

Brain and Nervous System: The brain comprises about 75% water, and proper hydration is vital for optimal function. Water helps cushion and protect the brain, regulates temperature, and facilitates the transmission of nerve impulses critical for cognitive processes and overall mental performance.

Muscles and Joints: Water is crucial for maintaining muscle function and joint lubrication. Proper hydration supports muscle contractions, helps prevent muscle cramps, and supports joint mobility by ensuring an adequate supply of synovial fluid, which cushions and lubricates the joints.

Digestive System: Water plays a vital role in digestion. It helps break down food, aids in nutrient absorption and supports the movement of waste through the gastrointestinal tract. It also helps prevent constipation by softening stools and promoting regular bowel movements.

What Happens When You Don't Drink Enough Water?

When dehydrated, the body's water balance is disrupted, leading to several physiological changes that can impair performance. Here are some effects of dehydration on mental and physical performance.

Mental Performance: Dehydration can impair cognitive abilities, including attention, concentration, and decision-making. It may lead to decreased alertness, difficulty focusing, and slower mental processing.

Did you know that dehydration can be the culprit behind those nagging headaches you get? When your body lacks sufficient fluids, it triggers a response from your brain that can lead to the constriction of blood vessels. This narrowing of blood vessels occurs as your body tries to regulate its fluid levels, and as a result, you may experience a headache.

Mood Changes: Dehydration can contribute to mood alterations, such as increased fatigue, irritability, and decreased motivation.

Physical Performance: Dehydration can negatively impact physical endurance, reducing stamina, increasing perception of effort, and decreasing exercise performance.

Impaired Temperature Regulation: Water plays a critical role in regulating body temperature through sweating. Dehydration can impair the body's ability to dissipate heat efficiently, potentially leading to overheating and an increased risk of heat-related illnesses.

Muscle Fatigue and Weakness: Inadequate hydration can result in muscle cramps, weakness, and decreased muscle coordination, which can affect overall physical performance and increase the risk of injuries.

Symptoms of dehydration can vary depending on the severity, but common signs include:

- Increased body temperature
- Headaches, Nausea or Dizziness
- Decreased blood pressure
- Excessive thirst
- Deterioration in concentration/cognitive function.

Determining optimal water intake depends on various factors such as age, sex, body weight, activity levels, and environmental conditions. A rough guide for adults is 2.1 litres per day for women and 2.6 litres for men.

Your urine colour is a simple and effective way to gauge hydration levels, with pale yellow indicating good hydration and darker shades signalling dehydration. However, remember that supplements like B vitamins, particularly B3 (niacin), can temporarily cause a bright yellow urine colour if consumed within 2–3 hours.

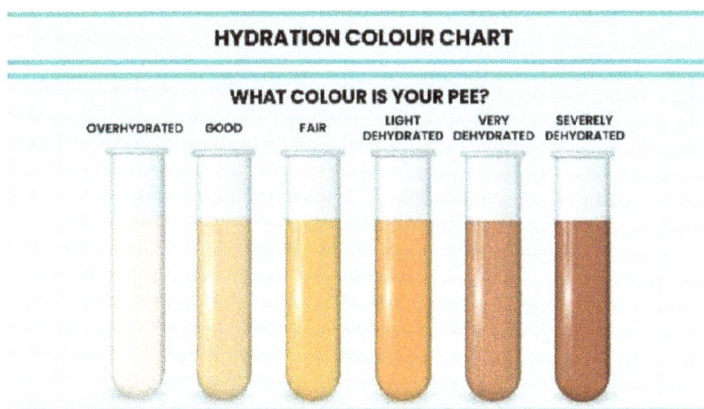

HYDRATION COLOUR CHART

WHAT COLOUR IS YOUR PEE?

| OVERHYDRATED | GOOD | FAIR | LIGHT DEHYDRATED | VERY DEHYDRATED | SEVERELY DEHYDRATED |

Hydration and Electrolytes for Peak Performance

Electrolytes are essential for maintaining optimal performance and health during play, training, or physically demanding activities. When you exercise, your body loses water and key electrolytes, such as sodium, potassium, calcium, and magnesium, primarily through sweat.

Electrolytes are vital for fluid balance, proper cell function, and key physiological processes such as muscular contractions, nerve signalling, and thermoregulation. Without adequate levels of electrolytes, your muscles, brain, and overall performance can suffer. Let's break down the recommended electrolytes and hydration guidelines based on exercise duration and intensity.

For Exercise Under 1 Hour (Low to Moderate Intensity):

Fluids: 200–400 ml of water during exercise may suffice, as electrolyte losses are typically minimal.

Electrolytes are unnecessary unless sweat loss is significant (e.g., in hot environments). A small amount of sodium can aid hydration.

For Exercise Over 1 Hour (Moderate to High Intensity):

Fluids: 400–800 ml of water per hour, adjusted for individual sweat rate and conditions.

Electrolytes: Sodium: 300–600 mg per hour to replace sweat losses and maintain fluid balance.

Potassium: 100–200 mg per hour to support muscle and nerve function.

For Intense Exercise Over 2 Hours or in Hot/Humid Conditions:

Fluids: 600–1,000 ml of water per hour, ideally combined with an electrolyte solution to maintain hydration and prevent hyponatremia (low sodium).

Electrolytes: Sodium: 500–1,000 mg per hour, depending on sweat loss.

Potassium: 150–300 mg per hour.

Magnesium: Small amounts, e.g. 50 mg per hour

Calcium: Minimal amounts, as calcium is less commonly lost in sweat, but it supports muscle function over longer durations.

Taurine – what is it, and why is it in everything?

I'm often asked why taurine is included in energy and electrolyte drinks. The answer lies in its versatile role in the body. Taurine is an amino acid that helps maintain fluid balance, supports energy production by optimising mitochondrial function, and aids muscle contractions through calcium regulation. It also protects cells with its antioxidant and anti-inflammatory properties, so overall, it is a very helpful ingredient.

Fuel To Thrive Nutritional Challenge

Level 1: Ditch the Junk - Eliminate highly processed food and drinks from your diet and replace them with healthier, nutrient-rich options.

If you feel anxious about giving up whatever unhealthy food you need, start by reducing the amount you consume for three days and then introduce a healthier option. Support this process by creating an environment that allows you to make the best choice.

Level 1.1: When you crave something that will prevent you from achieving your goals, practice 'Riding the Wave', which we discussed earlier.

Level 2: Plan and Prepare Home-Cooked Meals - Go and buy fresh produce from your local grocery store and prepare at least five evening meals during the week. Follow recipes or experiment with foods you like that align with your nutritional goals. Aim to include at least 20 different vegetables and fruits throughout the week. "I can't cook" will no longer be an excuse for eating out or getting takeaway.

Level 3: Calculate Your Caloric Needs - Start with your Basal or Resting Metabolic Rate (BMR) and then Estimate your Energy Requirement (EER). Now, establish your macronutrient breakdown and how much protein you need.

Level 3.1: Record all the food you eat using a food tracking app for one week to determine the quantity and quality of your nutritional intake.

Level 4: Supplement Smartly - If applicable to your goals, incorporate a suitable supplement into your routine.

Level 5: Hydration Habit - Track your water intake daily and ensure you meet or exceed the recommended hydration levels for your activity level.

Level 6: Performance Reflection - Reflect on how these dietary changes impacted your sleep, energy levels, mood, and overall performance throughout the week.

Pillar 4 - Personal Development and Mindset

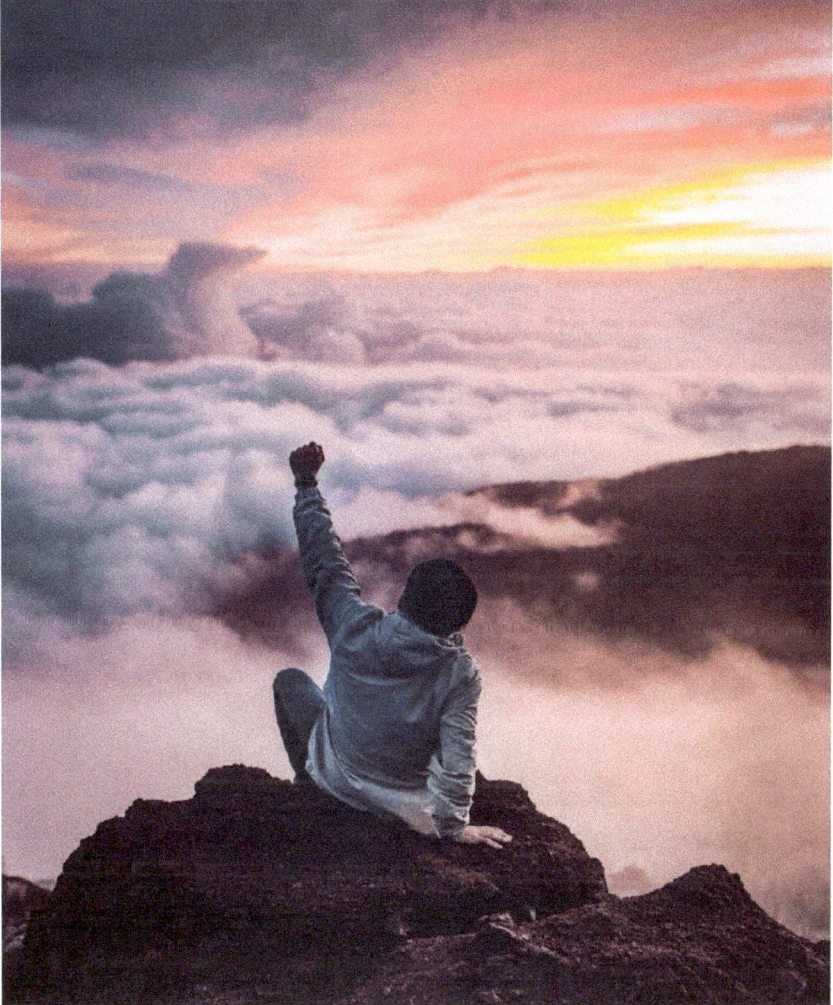

Part 1 - Unlocking Your Potential - Be The Best You Can Be!

The journey through adolescence into adulthood is one big developmental experiment. You start defining who you are, what you believe, and what you want to achieve in life.

These transitional years from teenager to adult are when we start to find our place in the world. However, very few people take the time to think about how they want their life to turn out. Whether you are 18 or 35, creating a clear vision of who you want to be and what your life will look like is essential. Please stop and think about it for 2 minutes and answer the following two questions.

What does your perfect life look like?

What does success look like for you?

A meaningful and fulfilling life should consist of a few fundamental components:

- Family
- Close friends
- Intimate relationships
- Educational goals
- Successful career
- Engaging time outside of work
- Attention to your mental and physical health

You may not need all of these things to have a rewarding and meaningful life, but you will need most of them!

Making decisive plans that will direct the next 5-10 years of your life can be overwhelming. However, with a well-thought-out plan for the future, you can avoid drifting through life, allowing external forces to shape your path rather than taking control of your destiny. It is very important to think about what you want in your life and how you want it to turn out. If you don't aim high, commit to something, or take on responsibilities, you will float along in a meaningless existence.

For young adults, investing in their mental and emotional maturity is important to achieving broader success and fulfilment in life. This is a pivotal stage in your life with endless potential and opportunities for growth, so it is important to visualise what you want to achieve in those fundamental areas.

Mental maturity is essential for navigating the challenges and complexities of life. It involves developing emotional resilience, self-awareness, and the ability to handle adversity. Mental maturity goes beyond chronological age; it is a mindset that encompasses self-reflection, a willingness to learn from experiences, and a commitment to personal growth.

Having a vision for your life is crucial for not getting stuck on the hamster wheel and falling into a self-pity hole when things go wrong. The road to success is never a straight-forward journey, but your vision serves as a compass, guiding your decisions and actions. By envisioning the kind of person you want to become, the values you want to embody, and the impact you want to make in the world, you set a clear direction, and now you just need to find the way.

Well-defined goals should accompany your vision. Goals provide the direction and stepping stones needed for realising your vision. They give you a sense of purpose, motivation, and a roadmap to follow. Having clearly defined goals helps you stay focused and accountable for your progress. Setting goals is so important that the next section is dedicated to the process.

Taking on responsibilities will allow you to derive meaning and purpose. It involves aligning your actions with your values and contributing to something greater than yourself.

Meaning and purpose can be found through various avenues, such as loving relationships, pursuing passions, engaging in service to others, or positively impacting society. Creating meaning and purpose in your life becomes the driving force that propels you towards success and fulfilment. Inevitably, you will face challenges, loss, and setbacks, so it is important to have relationships, hobbies, and work that bring you purpose and help you get through the tough times.

People who think that learning and growth stop after high school are the fools who will be working shitty jobs or living off the government. Embrace personal growth, remain open to new experiences, and continuously challenge yourself. With the right mindset and a commitment to your development, you can shape your future and create a personally and professionally rewarding life.

Developing mental strength and maturity is a lifelong journey. Embrace the process, endure the ups and downs, and be patient with yourself. You may not be able to accomplish much in a week or month, but you will be amazed at what you can accomplish in three or five years of consistent effort.

Success

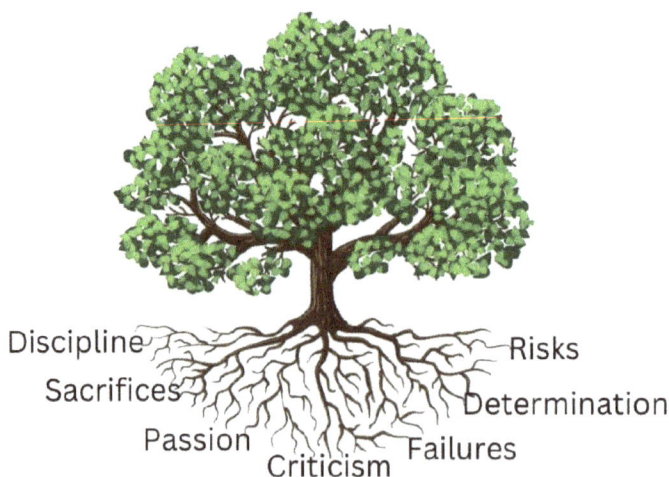

Discipline
Sacrifices
Passion
Criticism
Failures
Determination
Risks

Part 2 - Mindset Matters - How You View Things, Will Determine How You Do Things!

Your mindset plays a pivotal role in shaping your attitudes and behaviours and, ultimately, how you approach various aspects of life.

*Understand that how you **view** things will most likely determine how you do **things**!*

You will have to do things that don't excite you or are stressful and challenging. However, having the right mindset, such as a growth mindset or neutral thinking, can cultivate a mindset that will propel you towards success.

When approaching challenging or everyday tasks, you decide how much effort or focus you will give each activity. Don't underestimate the impact of repeated daily behaviours on your long-term success. Regardless of the activity, approaching it with the right mindset will help you navigate life and get the most out of yourself.

Growth Mindset - You Are Capable Of Anything

Life is an incredible journey full of twists, turns, and challenges. As you become a successful high performer, you'll encounter various obstacles and opportunities that will shape your future. But here's the secret sauce to conquering those challenges and continually adapting and growing - have a growth mindset!

Now, what exactly is a growth mindset? Well, it's the belief that your abilities and intelligence can be developed through effort, perseverance, and learning. It's about understanding that you have the power to improve, no matter your current position or where you have to start from. Imagine it as a superpower enabling you to face any challenge head-on and continue learning and improving. So, why is a growth mindset crucial for your success and well-being?

An excellent example of an athlete adopting a growth mindset is basketball legend Michael Jordan, one of my sporting heroes. Throughout his illustrious career, Jordan faced numerous challenges and setbacks, but his attitude and approach to those challenges set him apart.

In his sophomore year (10), Jordan was cut from his high school varsity team, a setback that could have discouraged many athletes. Instead of viewing this as a failure, Jordan saw it as an opportunity to grow. He used this setback as motivation to work harder and improve his skills.

Jordan didn't just bounce back; he thrived. He focused on continuous improvement by adopting a growth mindset and dedicated himself to developing his game. The following year, he made the varsity team and eventually went on to have one of the most successful careers in basketball history.

His growth mindset wasn't limited to overcoming setbacks. Jordan consistently sought opportunities to learn and refine his skills. Retiring from basketball to play baseball was a huge risk, but he saw an opportunity to challenge himself and develop a whole new set of skills. His work ethic and mindset were crucial in achieving six NBA championships and earning the title of one of the greatest basketball players ever.

Here Is How You Apply A Growth Mindset

Embracing Challenges: Instead of shying away from challenges, a growth mindset empowers you to welcome them with open arms. You see challenges as opportunities to learn and improve rather than threats to your self-worth. Embracing challenges helps you develop resilience and the confidence to tackle anything that comes your way.

Learning From Mistakes: We all make mistakes; it's part of being human. You understand that making mistakes is a natural part of the learning process, and they pave the way for growth and improvement. They are hard to deal with in the moment, but learning how to pick yourself up and keep improving will set you apart from your competitors.

FAILURE IS SIMPLY THE OPPORTUNITY TO BEGIN AGAIN,

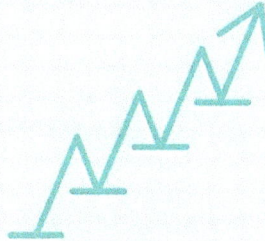

THIS TIME MORE INTELLIGENTLY.

Effort and Persistence: A growth mindset teaches you that effort and hard work are the keys to success. When faced with a difficult task, you don't give up easily. You're willing to put in the time and effort required to master new skills and achieve your goals.

Unleashing Your Potential: By adopting a growth mindset, you unlock your true potential. You break free from limiting beliefs and self-doubt, realising that your abilities are not fixed but can be cultivated and expanded with dedication and practice.

Lifelong Learning: Learning doesn't end with school or university; it's a lifelong journey. With a growth mindset, you're excited to continue learning and growing. Every experience, every challenge, and every new skill becomes an opportunity to evolve and become the best version of yourself.

Building Confidence: As you overcome challenges and witness your progress, your confidence soars. You start believing in your abilities and develop a strong sense of self-assurance. This self-belief becomes a powerful driving force in pursuing your dreams and aspirations.

Adopting a growth mindset doesn't mean you'll never face difficulties or doubts. It's about training your mind to see challenges as stepping stones, not stumbling blocks. It's about embracing the journey of learning and growth, knowing that every step you take brings you closer to success, no matter how small.

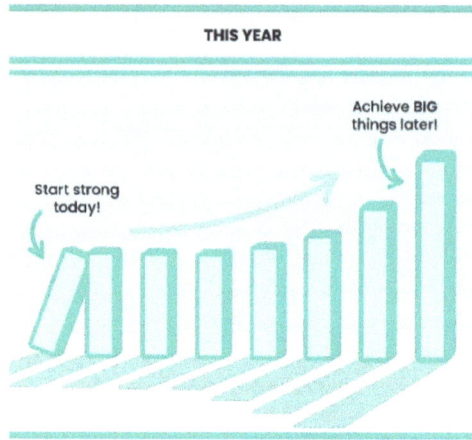

THIS YEAR

Achieve BIG things later!

Start strong today!

Adopting a growth mindset becomes a powerful starting point when facing challenging tasks. However, when you are in the moment, and things are not going according to plan, what can you do to keep moving forward?

Developing A Positive Mindset - Embrace The Power of Positivity

As you move through life, you will encounter many challenges and opportunities. Whether it's academic pressure, relationship issues, or personal goals, how you approach these challenges can make a significant difference in your overall well-being and success. One powerful tool at your disposal is adopting a positive mindset. Let's explore some excellent benefits of embracing positivity when facing life's hurdles.

Increased Resilience: Life is unpredictable, and setbacks are a natural part of the journey. A positive mindset helps you bounce back from disappointments and failures. Rather than getting bogged down by obstacles, you view them as opportunities for growth and learning. Resilience is a superpower that allows you to keep moving forward, no matter what comes your way.

Boosted Confidence: Confidence is the key to unlocking your potential. Embracing a positive mindset helps you build self-belief and trust in your abilities. Face challenges with positive optimism, knowing you can handle difficult situations.

Increased Motivation: Challenges can sometimes feel overwhelming, causing you to lose motivation. Remember, a positive mindset fuels your drive to persevere and gives you the strength to focus on your goals. It ignites your passion to keep striving for success, no matter how tough the road may seem.

Enhanced Problem-Solving Skills: A positive mindset fosters a "can-do" attitude, enabling you to approach challenges with creativity and resourcefulness. When you believe in your abilities to find solutions, you become more open to exploring different strategies and seeking help when needed. Problem-solving becomes an exciting adventure rather than an intimidating roadblock.

Remember, adopting a positive mindset doesn't mean you ignore reality or suppress negative emotions. It's about acknowledging the challenges yet responding with optimism and hope. Cultivating positivity takes time and effort, but it's a skill that will serve you well throughout your life.

I want to add one last and rarely discussed mindset that applies to all the competitive people reading this book: the Winning Mindset.

Winning Mindset

Once you learn how to win, it becomes a habit - a second nature that kicks in when it matters most. Think about Michael Jordan, Jonathan Thurston, Rafael Nadal or Michael Phelps. These athletes embody the Winning Mindset. They're the ones who win the big points or their teammates look to when the game is on the line. Why? Because they know how to focus in and get the job done, even when the odds are against them.

A winning mindset is more than just the desire to succeed; it's a finely tuned combination of self-belief, situational awareness, and adaptability. It's not enough to want to win - you must believe, deep down, that you have what it takes to come out on top, no matter the odds. This mindset separates those who get participation ribbons from those who consistently deliver results when it matters most.

Belief in your abilities is the cornerstone of the winning mindset. You need to think you're better than everyone else, not out of arrogance, but from a deep-seated confidence that you can execute when the clock is ticking and the pressure is on. You take ownership of the situation and execute on your skills. Self-belief and confidence enable you to perform under stress and make the right decisions in the heat of the moment.

But there's a critical difference between simply wanting to win and knowing how to win. The latter is a learned skill. It combines mastering your skill sets, mindset, and gameplay. You know you can break down opponents' strengths and weaknesses, evaluate and adapt on the move to refine your strategy and never stop coming at them. Some athletes become masters of this skill, knowing exactly how to secure a win even when their team is down or not at their best.

This winning mindset is about more than just wanting to win - it's about making winning a core part of who you are in every aspect of your life. This mindset makes you unrelenting in your pursuit of excellence, so much so that competitors dislike you for your intensity, and even teammates might find you challenging because you push them to their limits. You demand the best, both from yourself and those around you.

With a relentless focus on your goals and an unwavering commitment to excellence, you're willing to push beyond your comfort zone and make sacrifices to achieve greatness. Winning isn't just the outcome; it's a lifestyle and a personal standard that defines everything you do. You are willing to push to your limits and adopt a relentless focus on your goals and an unwavering commitment to excellence.

Once winning becomes a habit, it permeates every challenge you face. You're not just prepared for success in one area; you're equipped to excel across the board and turn opportunities into victories. You must think like a winner to be a winner.

Cultivating the right mindset has many benefits. However, when things are not going your way, having well-rehearsed behaviours to manage high-pressure situations. Knowing what they are and practising them so they are ready to use can be the difference between winning and losing.

Tools To Manage High-Pressure Performance Situations

Neutral Thinking - Focus On The Next Play.

Life can be like a rollercoaster ride, with exhilarating highs and challenging lows. When you face those tough moments, neutral thinking is a great technique for staying cool, calm, and focused.

So, what exactly is neutral thinking? Well, it's like slipping on a pair of 3D glasses that allow you to see situations from all angles with an unemotional, unbiased view. When you encounter a challenging moment, instead of getting overwhelmed by emotions, take a step back, breathe and look at the situation objectively.

Here's How You Can Implement Neutral Thinking

1. **Stay Present:** Focus on the present moment rather than getting caught up in what has just happened or the mistakes that occurred. You need to analyse the situation without any emotional bias and figure out what needs to be done next so you can respond effectively.

2. **Acknowledge Emotions:** It's essential to acknowledge your emotions without letting them overwhelm you. Recognise how you feel, but don't let strong emotions dictate your actions or cloud your judgement.

3. **Observe Without Judgement:** Look at the situation like a good commentator does: observe, analyse, and offer an opinion with minimal judgment. For example, how did that happen? What is going wrong? Who is playing well, who isn't, and why? What is the next play? How do I/we win from here?

By staying neutral, you don't get overwhelmed by what has just happened. You analyse the situation, accept what happened, and then plan for what you need to do next to achieve a better outcome.

Instead of dwelling on what went wrong or feeling overwhelmed by things you can't change, focus on what you can control. Constructive thoughts are much better than destructive thoughts. Here is an example of neutral thinking.

What can I do right now to help my team win the next play, improve my performance, or change the outcome of my situation?

Remember, feeling emotions is normal, but staying neutral helps you manage them effectively. It prevents knee-jerk emotional reactions and empowers you to respond thoughtfully and confidently. Whether it's a big performance, a missed goal on game day or a confrontational situation, staying focused and in control is your secret weapon, and the more you use it, the better you get at it. So, the next time you encounter a challenging situation, take a deep breath, put on those 3D glasses, and let Neutral Thinking guide you.

Change Your Voice: Inside vs. Outside

A group of scientists found that coping statements are more effective when verbalised. Inner talk is cognitively more sophisticated, so reverting to external dialogue can ease the burden and deliver a more concise and actionable message. Speaking out loud can help clarify thoughts and make coping strategies more effective, especially under stress. Another reason external self-talk can work well is that it holds you accountable to whoever is in earshot. This doesn't mean we should walk around saying all our thoughts aloud, but it might be a way to reach your overwhelmed brain that needs to pay attention and stop freaking out.

Decrease the Emotional Bond: From 'Me to 'You'

When we use third-person pronouns or our name, we create space between our sense of self and the situation. We transform into that friend who gives advice, not blinded by our connection to the issue.

According to researchers from the University of Michigan, first-person pronouns, e.g., I and me, tend to create a self-immersed world, while using words and phrases that create space produces a self-distanced perspective. When we can let go of the emotionality of the experience, we create psychological distance, which is often needed to refocus and tough it out. Self-immersed perspectives cause us to see the situation as a threat. When we adopt a self-distanced perspective, our views of the situation broaden.

We can let go of the emotions and see the situation for what it is rather than let it spiral - this is neutral thinking at work!

By creating this psychological distance, you can tackle the problem more strategically and clearly. So, instead of saying, "I can do this," I might say, "Josh, you've got this. Just stay focused and keep going." This self-distanced approach helps overcome the emotional bond connected to what just happened and improves the effectiveness of your self-talk and performance by keeping your thoughts composed and better directed.

Know What Voice to Listen To

It is often assumed that the way to better performance is through positivity, crowding out the doubts and negative emotions with words of affirmation and positive self-talk. There is plenty of evidence supporting this. However, a study on positive self-talk at the University of Waterloo found that positive self-talk worked as long as the subjects had high self-esteem. If they had low self-esteem, positive self-talk could be detrimental. In other words, your brain will not be fooled by false bravado. When it comes to self-talk, you won't make it if you fake it.

Imagine this: You're an athlete competing in a big event. You are trying to pump yourself up with positive self-talk, "You're the best, you can do this!" But what if, inside, you're struggling with self-doubt? Research suggests this kind of positive talk can backfire if you have low self-esteem.

Now, think about how negative self-talk fits into this. Some research shows that while excessive negative self-talk can be harmful, some can be helpful when used constructively and viewed as a motivational tool. The key is balance. If negative self-talk becomes overwhelming and affects your mindset, it's detrimental. However, if it's used sparingly and as a way to address areas of improvement, it can be beneficial. It's all about how you frame and balance your inner dialogue.

Many winners, whether in sports or other high-pressure scenarios, will use negative self-talk but tend to use it less and interpret what they say in a way that benefits them.

Psychologist Judy Van Raalte's research on tennis players found that winners and losers didn't differ in how much positive self-talk they used but noted that winners used less negative self-talk. However, when they dug into the data, they found that it wasn't so much whether some used positive or negative self-talk but how they interpreted it. Those who believed in their self-talk lost fewer points than those who saw it as irrelevant.

It's not just about what you say to yourself but how real it feels and how closely it aligns with your real-world performance. Know that both positive and negative self-talk can be useful, but pay attention to when it feels empty or detrimental and get better at using language that achieves the desired outcome.

The Power Of Negative Language: How Our Words Shape Our Outcomes

How we talk to ourselves and others can profoundly impact our personality and perception of reality. Our brains constantly listen to the language we use, whether it's our self-talk or the conversations we have with others. Just like a computer, our brains process and store information based on the software programs that are installed.

The words we use become the code our brains interpret and act upon. If we consistently use negative or self-defeating language, our brains will internalise those messages and start to create patterns of behaviours that align with those words.

For example, I often hear people say things like "I'm bad with names" or "I can never get this right," and guess what? They are right. They won't remember your name, and they always fail at simple problem-solving tasks.

Your brain will take those words as instructions and create the reality that matches those statements. Our brains are wired to seek evidence confirming our beliefs, and our language can reinforce those beliefs, especially when limiting or negative.

POWER VS BELIEF

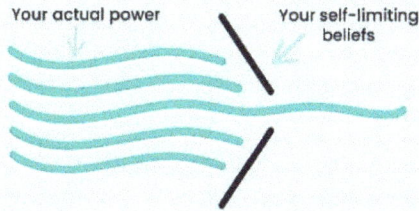

Your actual power

Your self-limiting beliefs

On the other hand, if you use empowering language such as "I will remember their name" or "I will try my best," your brain will interpret those words positively and increase your self-belief and subsequent performance.

It's not just about the words we use externally but also the words we use internally when we talk to ourselves. Our self-talk can profoundly impact our self-esteem, self-confidence, and overall well-being. If we consistently use negative or self defeating language, we are programming our brains to believe those negative messages. This will eventually manifest in our actions, behaviours and attitudes towards ourselves and others.

So, how can we use the power of language to shape our reality in a positive and empowering way?

1. **Be Mindful Of Your Language:** Pay attention to the words you use in your self-talk and conversations with others. Are they empowering or limiting? Are they positive or negative? Being aware of your language is the first step in making positive changes.

2. **Choose Empowering Words:** Use words that uplift and empower you. Instead of saying, "I can't do this," try saying, "I'll do my best." Instead of saying, "I hate this," try saying, "This is tough, but I will keep trying." Using words that reflect a growth mindset and a positive attitude can help rewire your brain for success and happiness.

3. **Reframe Negative Statements:** When you catch yourself using negative language, reframe those statements into positive or neutral ones. Instead of saying, "I'm terrible at this," try, "I'm still learning and getting better." In everyday conversations, we often say, "I have to go do something," as if it's a burden when it's actually a choice we've made.

   Try shifting your language from "I have to go to training, work, school" to "I get to go to training, work, school." This simple change can significantly shift your mindset, reminding you that you are in control of your actions. By choosing proactive language over reactive language, you empower yourself to take charge of your experiences.

4. **Don't Say Stupid Shit Out Loud:** If you are in a game or performance situation and things are not going to plan, don't say stupid things that won't help the situation. This will disrupt everyone around you, take your focus off the game and seldom lead to a positive outcome. Keep your cool and stay in control of your language. My motto is, don't get angry, get even. Beat them on the scoreboard.

5. **Practice Self-Compassion:** It's crucial to show yourself compassion when things don't go as planned or when you make a mistake. I used to fall into the habit of berating myself whenever I didn't win or perform well - calling myself all sorts of negative names and spending days replaying my mistakes. Self-reflection is fine but beating yourself up is not only deflating but counterproductive. The next time you catch yourself in a cycle of self-criticism, pause and recognise that thinking like this doesn't serve you.

   Instead, reflect on what happened with the same kindness and empathy you would offer a friend. Remember, treating yourself with compassion isn't about ignoring mistakes - it's about learning from them without tearing yourself down.

Once you start paying attention to your language, you will see how powerful and influential it is on you and everyone you encounter.

Seeking Support And Guidance

No one should navigate through challenges alone. Every high performer has a support team, so it's important to understand the value of seeking support or guidance. It is OK to reach out to trusted individuals, such as teachers, parents, or coaches, who can provide advice or assistance.

Asking for help is a sign of strength, not weakness, and collaboration can lead to more effective outcomes. By creating a sense of community and support, you will feel more empowered to face challenges head-on.

Having a winning mindset and incorporating neutral thinking can significantly impact how you think, feel, and approach stressful situations. Remember, you get to choose your language and how you apply yourself in any given situation.

So, whenever you encounter a hurdle or setback, take a deep breath, stay neutral and remind yourself that you can overcome anything.

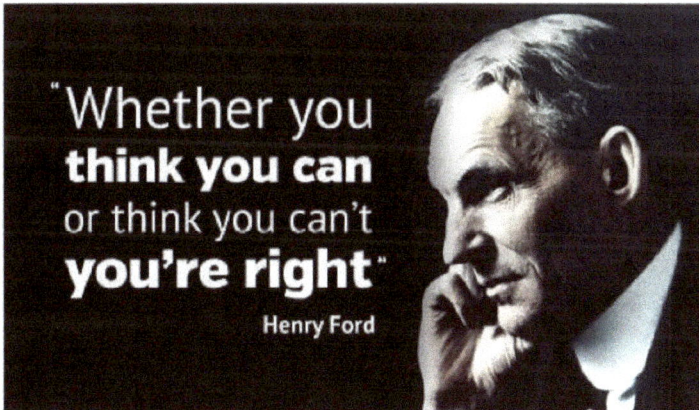

"Whether you **think you can** or think you can't **you're right**"

Henry Ford

Part 3 - Developing Leadership Skills: Unleashing The Leader Within

Developing leadership skills is important in a world full of opportunities and challenges. Whether leading a sporting or business team, managing family dynamics, or fostering personal growth, leadership qualities empower individuals to excel in various aspects of life.

We have all encountered good and bad leaders, and it doesn't take long to appreciate the qualities of a good leader. Leadership is underpinned by certain attributes or characteristics that influence behaviours and decision-making. These attributes are a set of trainable behaviours or traits that can be developed and utilised to optimise performance and navigate challenges effectively.

While personality traits might be relatively stable and inherent, attributes are more malleable and trainable. Individuals can develop and strengthen these attributes through intentional effort, practice, and experiences.

You hold the key to unlocking your potential as an effective leader in your journey of self-discovery and growth. Let's explore how you can become a leader in your personal, family, and professional life.

Leadership Qualities To Embrace

Inspiring and Visionary: Great leaders possess a clear vision and inspire others to rally around it. They communicate their vision effectively, painting a compelling picture of the future that motivates and energises their team or family. They ignite a collective drive towards shared goals by sharing their passion and purpose.

Authenticity - Be True to Yourself: Authenticity is the foundation of effective leadership. Embrace your unique qualities, values, and passions. Leaders who stay true to themselves inspire trust and create an environment where others feel comfortable being authentic. Reflect on your values, be transparent with your thoughts, and lead by example.

Authenticity fosters open communication and empowers your team to do their best.

Emotional Intelligence and Empathy: Leaders who bring out the best in others demonstrate emotional intelligence and empathy. They are attuned to the emotions and needs of those around them, actively listening and seeking to understand. By showing genuine care and concern, they foster a supportive environment where individuals feel valued, heard, and empowered to reach their full potential.

Effective Communication: Leadership thrives on effective communication. Skilful leaders excel at both expressing their ideas and actively listening to others. They communicate with clarity, transparency, and respect, ensuring that messages are understood and promoting open dialogue. By fostering effective communication, they create a collaborative and trusting atmosphere.

Trustworthiness and Integrity: Leaders who elicit the best from their team or family prioritise trust and integrity. They lead by example, consistently acting honestly, transparently, and fairly. Maintaining their integrity and keeping their commitments builds trust and credibility, fostering strong relationships and a positive work or family culture.

Coaching and Development: Exceptional leaders focus on their team members' growth and development. They act as coaches and mentors, supporting others' aspirations and providing guidance and opportunities for improvement. They unleash their potential by investing in their growth and cultivating a high-performance culture that drives collective success.

Adaptability and Resilience: Leaders who thrive in different contexts exhibit adaptability and resilience. They embrace change, navigate challenges with composure, and encourage others to view setbacks as opportunities for learning and growth. By modelling adaptability and resilience, they foster an environment encouraging innovation, agility, and continuous improvement.

Developing Your Leadership Behaviours - When And Where To Flex Those Leadership Muscles

Have you ever thought of yourself as a leader? No? Well, it's time to change that! Did you know leadership isn't just about being the loudest in the room or having a fancy job title? It's about influence. It's about inspiration. It's not confined to the boardroom or the battlefield. Leadership is a superpower we all have, and it can be applied in every aspect of our lives.

Leadership is not about superhuman feats – it's about using your abilities to positively shape those around you. It's about being a beacon of inspiration and a pillar of support.

Think about it. In your personal life, you can lead by example among your friends and social circles. You can be the one who organises fun gatherings, initiates important conversations, or stands up against injustice. You can inspire your siblings and relatives to reach their goals in your family. You can take the reins of projects or strategic initiatives in your professional life, leading confidently and gracefully.

Leadership: Much More Than a Buzzword

Remember, leadership isn't just a fancy buzzword. It's about influencing and inspiring others to be their best selves and doing so with humility and compassion. Always consider the needs and well-being of those you lead.

Imagine the transformative journey of developing these leadership skills as your career develops. The lifelong benefits that come with it are like a treasure chest waiting to be unlocked. And guess what? You hold the key!

When you wholeheartedly embrace a clear vision, demonstrate genuine empathy, communicate effectively, build trust, uplift others, and remain adaptable and resilient, you become the catalyst for growth and transformation. Like sunlight to a seedling, you nurture environments that foster the potential in everyone around you.

Everyone can cultivate these essential skills, but only a few do. Develop the leader within you, and get ready to see your career develop faster than those around you. The world needs effective and inspiring leaders, so shine brightly and lead with purpose.

Upgrade Your Mindset and Language Challenge

Level 1: Morning Mindset Challenge

Build this into your morning routine when your mind is most receptive. It will be the perfect time to set the tone for your day. You can include this in your breathwork, meditation or intention-setting practice.

Affirm Your Positivity: Begin by saying to yourself, "Today, I choose to be positive." This reminds you that positivity is a choice, not a reaction to circumstances. It sets the foundation for approaching challenges with optimism.

Practice Gratitude: Reflect on a few things you're grateful for, such as your health, loved ones, or opportunities. Gratitude shifts your focus from scarcity to abundance, creating a mindset of appreciation.

Set Your Intention: Decide how you want to show up for the day. To affirm your belief in your abilities, say, "I am capable of achieving great things. " Follow this with a specific intention, such as, "I will bring focus and effort to my tasks today."

Visualise Success: Take 1–2 minutes to visualise your day going well - seeing yourself overcoming obstacles, engaging positively with others, and progressing toward your goals.

Level 2: Language Makeover - Reframe your language

The next time you catch yourself using negative or unhelpful language - whether it's about a task, a person, or a situation - pause and take control. Instead of letting the negativity spiral, consciously reframe your words into positive or neutral statements. Avoid getting drawn into complaining or criticising things outside your control (your circle of concern). Shift your usual response from a reactive, negative comment to a thoughtful, constructive one.

Level 3: Neutral Thinking in Practice

When you are next in a high-pressure situation, e.g., a game, training, or performance situation, and things are not going your way, stop and apply neutral thinking. Break down the situation, analyse it calmly, acknowledge emotions, and reframe negative thoughts. Reflect on how your change in response improved your performance and the situation's outcome.

Level 4: Be The Leader

When an opportunity arises to step forward and lead the group, take on assignments or resolve issues, don't sit back and wait for someone else to take control.

Pillar 5 - Habits and Behaviours

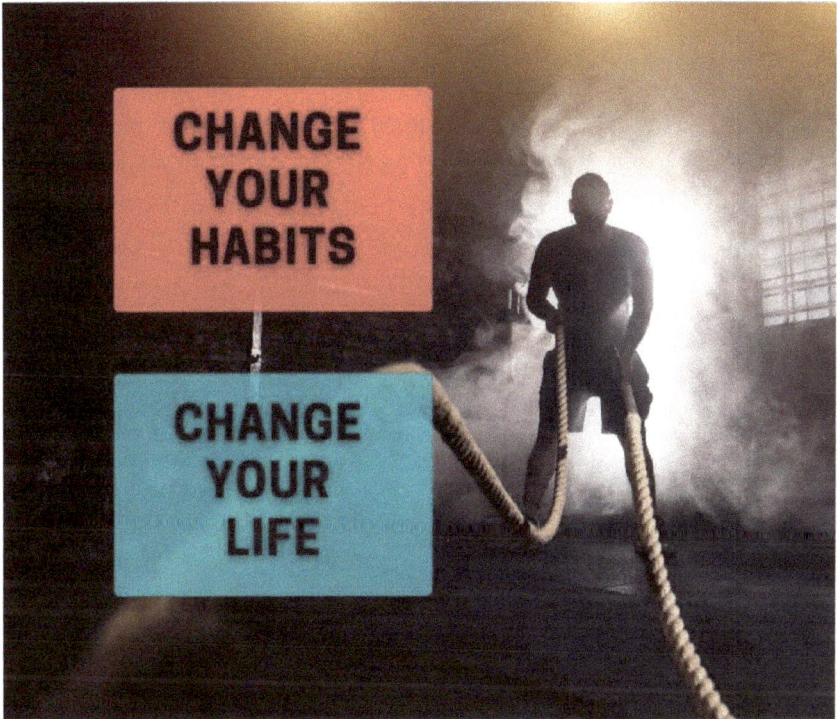

Part 1 - Goal Setting For A Better Future

What is the point of setting goals?

Just imagine sitting on a sailboat without a compass or navigation tools. You have no direction, no destination, and no purpose. That's life without goals! Goals are like the compass that guides your journey through life. They give you a sense of direction and purpose and motivate you to get out of your comfort zone.

You don't just set the goal to achieve it. You set the goal for who it will require you to become in the process of achieving it. It's about the journey, the preparation, the commitment, and the transformation. The goals must be big enough that you are excited by who they will require you to become. Even if you don't reach the end goal, you will have hit many milestones and grown as a person. This is the hidden reason why we need goals in our lives.

However, just jotting down any old goal is not enough. It's like saying, "I want to be a millionaire", without knowing how or when you will achieve that. You need a proper plan, a timeline, and a lot of determination to get there. So buckle up, and let's explore the fascinating world of goal setting!

In 1990, Professors Edwin Locke and Gary Latham published - A Theory of Goal Setting and Task Performance, where they identified the **five principles of effective goal setting.**

Clarity - Specific goals put you on a direct course. When a goal is vague, it has limited motivational value.

Commitment - refers to the degree to which an individual is attached to the goal and their determination to reach it, even when faced with obstacles.

Challenge - Goals must be challenging yet attainable. Challenging goals can improve performance through increased self-efficacy.

Task complexity - Overly complex goals that are beyond our skill level may become overwhelming and negatively impact morale, productivity, and motivation.

Feedback - Goal setting is more effective in the presence of external and internal feedback. This helps to determine the degree to which a goal is being met and how you are progressing.

Goal Setting: The Art And Science

Let's break the process into two systems. The first is outlining your vision and desired outcomes, and the second is creating the checkpoints and time frame in which you want them to happen. It's like baking a cake; you need a clear picture of what you want to bake, check that you have the right ingredients, and then work out the instructions(process) and time frame required to get a delicious result. Goal Setting is working backwards from what you want to achieve and outlining the method and ingredients needed to produce the perfect result.

Creating Your Recipe for Success: Define Outcome, Learning, Process, and Performance Goals

Like a chef preparing a three-course meal, we need to prepare and plan to ensure things are done in the right order and with the right ingredients. The goal-setting menu typically offers three types of goals: outcome, process, and performance goals. But I like to add a secret ingredient to this mix - a learning goal!

Outcome Goals: These are your big, hard goals. Like aiming for that dream job, playing sports professionally or losing 10kgs. They're the main course of your goal-setting menu.

Learning Goal: This is your foundation layer to achieving success. Just like you can't build a house without first laying a solid foundation, you can't accomplish a goal without first understanding the basics. It's like wanting to lose weight but not knowing which foods will support this goal. A better knowledge of the skill set, behaviour or rules empowers you to apply your best self to the situation. Understanding WHY things need to be done in a certain way produces better long-term outcomes.

Learning goals are the most overlooked component of effective goal setting because if you have a poor understanding of what is required, how will you set realistic and meaningful goals? If you are new to a goal arena or want to take your skill or behaviour to the next level, then building your knowledge in this space is important to your long-term success.

Performance Goals: These are the milestones or benchmarks you set to measure and track your progress toward the outcome goal.

Process Goals: these are the daily and weekly habits combined with your training and nutritional requirements needed to reach your performance and, ultimately, outcome goals.

If your outcome goal is to run a marathon, the process starts with running five kilometres four days a week, then eight kilometres and so on, continually hitting the performance goals needed to be ready for race day. To reach that big, challenging goal, it's essential to establish all the right behaviours, strategies, and training routines.

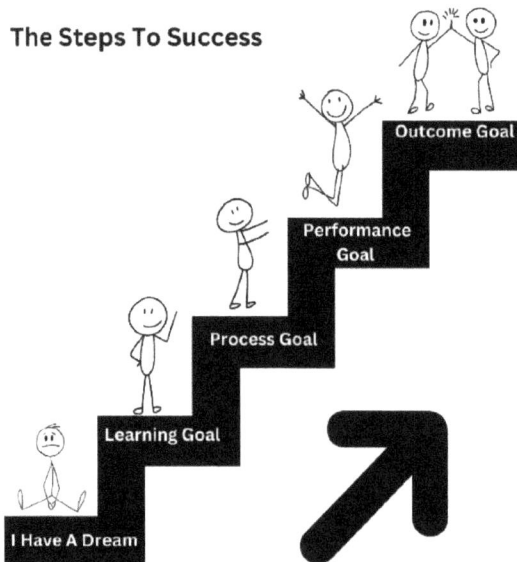

The Steps To Success

- Outcome Goal
- Performance Goal
- Process Goal
- Learning Goal
- I Have A Dream

Breaking Down Your Goals: Clarity Equals Confidence

Have you ever tried reaching a destination without knowing where it is? Sounds absurd, right? That's why it's crucial to visualise your future. Imagine what your best life looks like, what you want to achieve, and what makes you feel fulfilled. But remember, every goal comes with a price. Are you ready to sacrifice your Netflix binge for that study or workout session?

Once your goals are clear, you can break them down into smaller, manageable steps. This helps you create a roadmap to your destination. And remember, the clearer your goals, the easier it is to track your progress and make necessary adjustments.

Finally, remember that goal setting is just the start. The real challenge is sticking to your plan, and to do this, you need to create systems in your life that support your goals and allow you to stay committed to your journey, even when things get tough.

"You don't rise to the heights of your goals; you fall to the level of your systems" - James Clear.

Goal Setting - Let's Do It The Right Way

Step 1: Establish Outcome Goals = Long-Term Goal

This is your massive transformative goal. What do you want to achieve in your life over the next 1, 3, or 5 years? Identify your big, hard goals and then work backwards from there.

Step 2: Identify Learning Goals

Review your goal arena (skill, sport, behaviour etc) and identify where you need to increase your skills, knowledge and understanding of what is required to be successful. Create learning goals that can integrate into your process and performance goals.

Ask yourself: Do you have a good understanding of the rules, skills, and strategies? What is the best equipment? How should I be training? How can I improve my recovery? Do you know what the best people in your field are doing to succeed?

Outline what you need to know to improve your chance of success and include them in your process goals. Integrate your learning goals into your new habits as part of your process goals.

Step 3: Create Performance Goal = Medium-Term Goals

These are the tokens you need to collect to get to the next level, and they can take months or years to accomplish. They are the milestones, e.g., wins, PBs, goals, qualifications, performances, etc, required to achieve the big hard goal from Step 1. They should be challenging but attainable and direct what you need to do weekly. They need to have a time frame on them as well.

Step 4: Outline The Process Goals = Short-Term Goals

What are you doing daily to move you closer to the performance goals you have set for yourself in Step 3? It is super important to set clear daily and weekly goals. They can range from daily habits, training sessions, meal times, bedtime routines or behaviours that will help you move forward and be successful.

Example Of Goal Setting Process: Playing Cricket For Australia

Step 1:Setting the Big Hard Goal = Outcome Goal

My big, hard goal is to play cricket for the Australian national team in 3 years. This is my ultimate dream, and it will be the driving force behind the entire goal-setting process.

Step 2: Lay the Foundations = Learning Goal

I'm 17 years old and representing my region at the state championships. My learning goal is to understand the selection process, who the selectors are, what they are looking for, and who I will play against. I will also find out if I can attend training camps to develop my skills and ensure I do the right things to become a professional cricket player.

Step 3: Markers To Measure Progress = Performance Goals

I use my yearly planner to break down my sports season or performance calendar. I establish how many weeks I have to prepare and when I am competing, and then I set my performance goals.

1. Improve my batting average by 20 runs by the Christmas break = 50 runs per innings.

2. Play in the Wide Bay rep team at the state championship in January. Get at least two 50+ run scores while playing at number 3.

3. Get selected for the Queensland U18 team and attend the national championships tournament in February.

Step 4: Create The Map For Success = Process Goals

I will create a tailored exercise program that aligns with my team's training plan and outlines my daily habits. The following is just an example, your plan should contain more details.

Monday - 30-minute jog and weight session in the gym.

Tuesday - Team net session

Wednesday - HIIT session and fielding practice.

Thursday - Team Net Session

Friday - 40-minute jog and mobility work.

Saturday - Game

Sunday - Rest or 30-minute walk on the beach

Step 5: Review And Seek Feedback On Your Progress

Reviewing and seeking feedback is not just a reflection process but a dynamic part of your journey towards hitting your goals. It empowers you to make informed decisions, stay motivated, and continually optimise your training and behaviours for optimal results.

Where Is The SMART Goal Setting?

Why are SMART goals all you hear about when it comes to goal setting? Originally, SMART goals were designed from a corporate perspective and can be useful in certain environments. However, in my experience, using the SMART acronym does not work when it comes to personal growth or behaviour change.

The SMART acronym was first documented in 1981 by the former Director of Corporate Planning for Washington Water Power Company. It was published in a paper titled "There's a S.M.A.R.T. Way to Write Management's Goals and Objectives."

Too often, people fill in the S, M, A, R, and T but don't follow through and outline the important details - the short, medium, and learning goals needed to create an actionable plan. The goal lacks clarity and an understanding of the commitments needed to reach the desired outcome. That is why so many goals go unattained and why I recommend the four-step process outlined above.

Staying Committed - The Real Challenge

Embarking on a journey to success demands more than just crafting a plan - it's about wholeheartedly embracing and sticking to it. Creating a straightforward plan you can commit to surpasses any convoluted strategy that is too hard and will be abandoned two weeks in.

Stay committed to your goals by creating an environment that supports your journey to success. This involves creating a structured training schedule, seeking mentorship or coaching, and maintaining a balanced lifestyle that aligns with your goals.

Remember, achieving your dreams requires hard work, dedication, and sacrifice. Even when faced with challenges, keep pushing forward with determination and passion.

Following a goal-setting process and creating a clear roadmap can lead to extraordinary accomplishments. But most people I know, myself included, have set goals that have gone unaccomplished.

Why does this happen? It could be due to not regularly reviewing and adjusting your goals or staying disciplined in your training and preparation. It can be various things, but evidence suggests that failures arise from not establishing the right systems in your day-to-day environment. Systems are your daily processes, routines, and habits for achieving your goals. Creating clear goals is essential for setting a direction, but systems are what lead to progress and success.

How To Achieve Your Goals Consistently

Practical goal setting requires considering the environment and systems you need to implement. Too often, we set the right goals inside the wrong system. Without the right systems in place, it will be hard to make consistent progress.

All kinds of hidden forces make our goals easier or harder to achieve. You need to align your environment with your ambitions to see success in the long run. Let's discuss some practical strategies for doing just that.

Align Your Environment With Your Goals

The environment you work and live in is an invisible glove that shapes your behaviour. We tend to believe our habits are a product of our motivation, talent, and effort. Certainly, these qualities matter. But the surprising thing is that your personal attributes tend to get overpowered by your environment. Although most of us can make a wide range of choices at any given moment, we often make decisions based on the environment we find ourselves in. Do not underestimate the importance of creating an environment where you can do your best work.

For example, if I wanted to, I could drink a beer as I write this book. However, I sit at my desk with a glass of water next to me. There are no beers in sight. It is essential to set your environment up so it is easy to make the best decisions and keep you on the right path to achieving your goals.

Here are some examples of how the environment will direct your behaviours.

If you sleep with your phone next to your bed, you will find it hard to stop scrolling or chatting when it is time to sleep. Then, the first thing you do when you wake up is to check your phone for notifications or emails, which is the opposite of what you should be doing to start the day.

If you walk into your bedroom and you have a TV on the wall, you will most likely watch some pointless show rather than wind down with a book and go to sleep.

If you keep soft drinks, sweets and cakes in your kitchen, then consistently snacking on unhealthy treats is more likely to be the default decision.

Let's flip this to the positive side so it helps make the right decision easy.

You install a smart plug that turns off the Wi-Fi at 9 p.m., so you are not tempted to keep watching Netflix or scrolling Instagram.

Fresh fruit is on the bench, and a bag of mixed nuts is in the cupboard. You carry a water bottle throughout the day, so drinking water becomes easy and the default decision.

You set a bedtime reminder, prepare your training gear, and then go to bed to allow for an 8-hour sleep window so you are well-rested and ready for the early morning training session.

Scientists refer to the impact of environmental conditions on our decision-making as choice architecture. Whether or not you achieve your goals in the long term has a lot to do with the types of influences, both environmental and people surrounding you in the short term. It's tough to stick with positive habits in an unsupportive environment. Create an environment to facilitate the right choice being made.

Strategies To Create Better Systems In Your Life

Remove Temptation: Removing temptations is a powerful way to design an environment that supports your goals and minimises distractions. Eliminating obstacles and reducing access to negative influences makes it easier to focus, stay consistent, and achieve success. Here are examples to apply this strategy effectively:

Healthy Eating:

- Remove junk food from your pantry and replace it with nutritious snacks like nuts, fruit, and yogurt.

- Prepare your meals in advance to avoid eating unhealthy takeout or fast food when you're busy or tired.

Productivity:

- Turn off non-essential notifications on your phone and computer to avoid constant interruptions.

- Use tools like website blockers (e.g., Freedom, Focus) to prevent access to distracting websites during work hours.

- Create a clutter-free workspace with only the essentials to help you concentrate.

Financial Habits:

- Unsubscribe from retail email lists to resist impulse buying and avoid unnecessary temptations.

- Automate savings by setting up direct transfers to a savings account before you can spend the money.

Fitness and Exercise:

- Join a Gym Near Your Home or Work: Make getting to the gym as convenient as possible, reducing the temptation to skip workouts.

- Set a Fixed Workout Schedule: Block out time on your calendar for exercise, just like you would for an important meeting. This removes the decision-making process and reduces excuses.

- Schedule Workouts in the Morning: Exercise first thing in the day to avoid the temptation of skipping after work due to fatigue or other commitments.

Social Media Use:

- Log out of social media apps after use, or set time limits using built-in tools on your device.

- Delete apps from your phone if they're a persistent distraction, and access them only on a computer at designated times.

Sleep:

- Remove screens from your bedroom and replace them with books or relaxation tools, such as a journal or guided meditation app.

- Set your phone to "Do Not Disturb" mode and place it across the room to avoid late-night scrolling.

Visual Cues: Create a visual habit tracker, whether a physical chart on your wall or a digital one on your device. Mark it off each time or day you complete the desired behaviour. Visual progression over time is a motivating and rewarding cue that reinforces the habit. This relates back to - what gets measured, gets managed.

Opt-Out vs. Opt-In: A famous organ donation study revealed how multiple European countries skyrocketed their organ donation rates by requiring citizens to opt-out rather than opt-in. You can do something similar in your life by creating systems that make committing to the desired behaviour easier.

For example, you could sign up and pay for the upcoming health retreat weeks in advance, buy a three-month coaching package, register for a class when you feel motivated, etc. Committing to something or someone provides accountability and makes it hard to opt out when the time comes because you are letting down not only yourself but also someone else and probably losing money as well.

Create a Support Network: Tell the important people in your life what you want to achieve and explain the time commitments and training it will take. This firstly creates accountability but also outlines when you will be around to help out or socialise and when you will need their support or absence so you can do your thing.

The Illusion Of Choice: Commitments And Sacrifice

Chasing big, hard goals can often limit the life choices you get to make. If you want to be successful as an athlete or high performer, you automatically lose the ability to choose to do many things.

For example, practising your skills 10+ hours a week becomes mandatory, so you lose the choice to watch 2-3 hours of TV in the evening, go to a party or hang out with friends all the time. Because you are training so hard, you need to make sure you are doing the recovery sessions and getting enough good quality sleep, so to do this, you go to bed early enough to get 7-8 hrs sleep and don't drink alcohol during the week, or at all.

When you choose to pursue a goal and are serious about it, many of your decisions are now made for you, which is great for people who can't say no.

Achieving great things requires hard work and sacrifice. But if you have a strong enough WHY, you will overcome any HOW! This is why you need a clear vision and purpose for your future. Recognising the significance of seemingly small daily decisions and subsequent behaviours is essential. They may only take a few minutes or seconds, but add them up over time, and you realise it was worth getting them right. These daily decisions may not appear all that important, but they are directly related to producing the results we want in the long run.

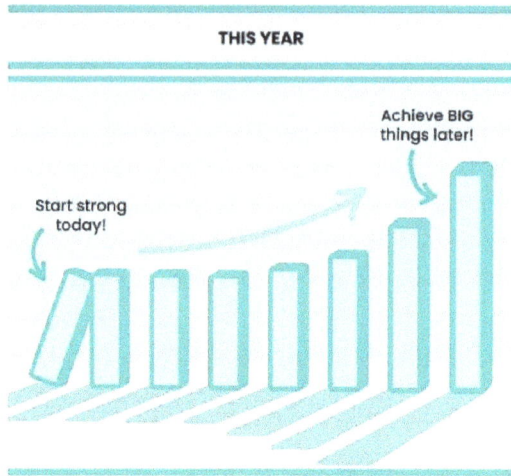

Embrace the value of consistency and realise that even the smallest actions will contribute to your long-term success. Committing to continuous improvement and being willing to overcome setbacks will lay the foundation for achieving great things.

Understand that each investment you make in yourself, no matter how minor, has the potential to compound over time. Much like the power of compound interest in finance, these daily efforts and sacrifices accumulate and pave the way to success.

How To Know You Are Moving In The Right Direction - Measure Your Progress

How do you know you are getting better and moving in the right direction? Measurement and Feedback. The human mind loves to receive feedback, and one of the most motivating things we can experience is evidence of our progress. This is why measurement is so critical for achieving goals. By measuring or tracking your results, you get insights into whether you are progressing or not.

However, the trick is not to get emotionally manipulated or consumed by the numbers. Sometimes, they are not what you want to see or don't give you a true indicator of how you feel. We must be able to step back and reflect on all the other areas of our lives that contribute to achieving our goals. Just because you got a bad sleep score, didn't get the time you wanted, or missed a lift at the gym doesn't mean your day is ruined and everything will be lost.

Identify the few key activities, exercises, or behaviours that drive the majority of your success. This is the essence of the 80/20 Pareto Principle: in any pursuit, a small number of contributors often account for the largest impact.

Track what brings the most significant results and helps you stay consistent in your training. Since we can't measure everything, focus on what gives you the most valuable feedback to stay motivated, avoid burnout, and prevent injury. Remember, listening to your body's signals is essential. It's always providing feedback on how you're progressing.

Here are three key areas an athlete could focus on and track:

Performance Metrics: These could include time trials, speed, power output, agility tests, strength levels, or skill-specific metrics like shooting accuracy or technical proficiency.

Recovery Metrics: Monitoring sleep quality, heart rate variability (HRV), and resting heart rate can help you understand how well you're recovering from training and competition, which is crucial for sustained performance.

Nutrition and Hydration: Tracking your dietary intake, including macronutrients, hydration levels, and any supplements, ensures your body is getting the fuel it needs to perform and recover optimally.

Part 2 - Exploring Habits - How To Start New Habits And Stop Bad Ones.

Let's explore the underpinning aspects of achieving our goals - our habits and behaviours and the systems that keep us accountable. When I finally understood the science behind our everyday behaviours, it changed how I looked at making changes and coaching people to achieve better outcomes. Equipping yourself with the knowledge of how to start new habits, kick those unwanted ones, and establish the right systems will skyrocket your health and performance.

Setting goals is pretty straightforward. The real test lies in implementing the behaviours alongside the sacrifices required to achieve them. After all, a goal is only as effective as the system or set of behaviours it operates on. Creating systems is crucial to performing at your best over the long term. Step one in learning to stop unwanted habits is understanding what drives our behaviours.

The Habit Loop - Cue, Craving, Response, Reward

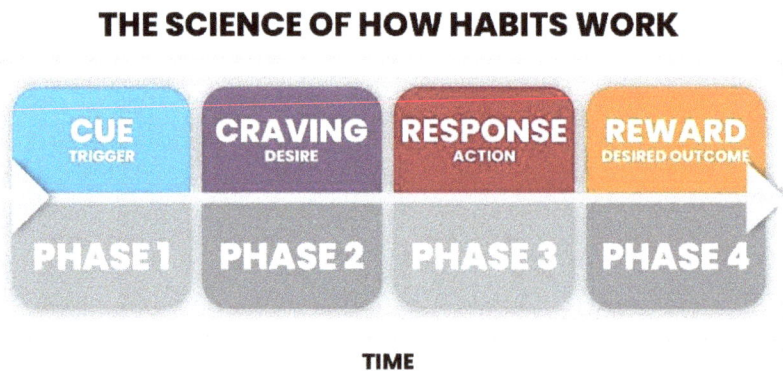

THE SCIENCE OF HOW HABITS WORK

CUE TRIGGER	CRAVING DESIRE	RESPONSE ACTION	REWARD DESIRED OUTCOME
PHASE 1	PHASE 2	PHASE 3	PHASE 4

TIME

Understanding the habit loop can be a powerful tool for achieving your goals. Recognising that every action begins with a trigger allows you to shape an environment that supports the choices you want to make. By identifying what triggers your cravings or actions, you gain insight into why you respond in certain ways, often in pursuit of a specific outcome.

Whether you're studying for an exam or aiming to elevate your performance on the track or field, mastering this loop gives you the control to steer your habits in any direction you choose. And there's even more beneath the surface to explore.

Our brains are sophisticated prediction machines. When we experience something good, favourable, or pleasurable, our brain marks that experience with a positive chemical signal - often dopamine. This chemical reward signals that something valuable has occurred, and our brain takes note. The next time we encounter a similar situation, our brain predicts that the same positive outcome is possible, driving us to seek that experience again. This prediction and reward system is why habits can become so deeply ingrained. The brain isn't just reacting to the present; it's predicting the future based on past experiences.

When you understand this mechanism, you gain the power to shape your habits consciously. By recognising the triggers that lead to the rewarding behaviours, you can reinforce positive habits that propel you toward your goals or rewire negative ones that hold you back. By mastering the habit loop, you're not just changing what you do - you're retraining your brain to predict and crave the outcomes that lead to your success.

1. Cue: This is your starting point, the trigger that signals your brain to take action. It could be a thing or place, a time, an emotion, a person, or an alert. It is a bit of information that sets the behaviour in motion. Identify the cue, and you're on your way.

2. Craving: This is the motivational force that drives the behaviour, getting you to act. Think of it as the voice saying, "Hey, wouldn't it be awesome if you did this right now? It was good last time."

3. Response: It's the action, behaviour, or routine you go through to get the desired outcome your brain or stomach is seeking. This could be hitting the gym, buying ice cream, picking up your phone to scroll social media, or eating a healthy or unhealthy meal.

4. Reward: This is where the behaviour is reinforced or rejected. Through emotions and feelings, a feedback loop is established. If there is a positive outcome, your brain records it as something worth doing again, and then this reinforces the craving in the process next time. The cues and cravings set the behaviour in motion, and regardless of whether it is adaptive or maladaptive, the habit has happened and is rewarded.

This habit loop is not an occasional occurrence but an ongoing feedback loop that happens subconsciously throughout the day. The brain is in constant motion, scanning the environment, anticipating future events, experimenting with various responses, and assimilating lessons from the outcomes. This entire cycle unfolds within seconds, and we engage in it repeatedly, often without full awareness. Now you know how habits work, let's turn this information into a framework to help you create positive new habits.

Creating New Habits

Starting a new habit or behaviour can be challenging, so you need to use the right tactics to move the needle in your favour. James Clear has developed a framework called the Four Laws of Behaviour Change, which, when applied correctly, can be a game changer.

Each law is a lever that can be pulled to increase the chance of the behaviour becoming a habit and you making long-term changes.

How to Create a Good Habit	
The 1st law (Cue)	**Make it Obvious**
The 2nd law (Craving)	**Make it Attractive**
The 3rd law (Response)	**Make it Easy**
The 4th law (Reward)	**Make it Satisfying**

Here is an example of how the four laws can be applied to starting a new 30-minute morning walk or exercise routine.

Make it Obvious (Cue): Place your shoes, socks and outfit near your bed the night before. Seeing these items as soon as you wake up is a visual cue, that you need to go for your morning walk/workout.

Make it Attractive (Craving): Choose a scenic route for your walk, play your favourite podcast or music during the walk or invite a friend to join you. Making the walk enjoyable and appealing increases your craving for this positive experience.

Make it Easy (Response): Not only will you have your walking gear ready the night before, but you will also go to bed early enough so you wake up on time, feeling refreshed and ready to go. The easier it is to get up and go, the more likely you will follow through.

Make it Satisfying (Reward): After completing your morning walk, treat yourself to a nutritious breakfast and a cup of coffee. The sense of accomplishment coupled with a satisfying reward reinforces the behaviour, making it more likely to become a habit.

Stopping Bad Habits

Breaking free from unwanted habits might seem simple; you just need to invert the Four Laws of Behaviour Change. But if it were easy, why do so many of us still struggle to stop behaviours that harm our health and performance? The answer lies in understanding how the brain works and how addictive behaviours exploit the scarcity loop, a concept explored in Michael Easter's book, *Scarcity Brain*. His work highlights why some habits are so hard to quit - they hi-jack our brain's primal wiring.

Until relatively recently, most resources, such as food, shelter, and safety, were scarce and required work to obtain. Our ancestors evolved to seek out every possible opportunity to secure these resources, investing energy in pursuits that might yield rewards. If a tactic failed, they'd adapt and repeat their efforts to increase their odds of a positive outcome. This scarcity-driven survival instinct kept our ancestors alive, but in today's world of abundance, it is working against us. The same impulses that helped our ancestors survive now lock us into behaviours we struggle to control.

The scarcity loop sits at the heart of many of our hardest-to-break habits. It's a cycle driven by three elements: **opportunity, unpredictable rewards, and quick repeatability**. Recognising this loop is essential to dismantling it:

1. **Opportunity**: The more accessible a behaviour is, the more likely you are to repeat it. Think of social media on your phone, an endless scroll of opportunities to be entertained and stimulated at your fingertips. Each notification presents a chance to engage with the app, and the ease of access makes it hard to resist.

2. **Unpredictable Rewards**: We're drawn to behaviours with uncertain rewards because unpredictability triggers a powerful release of dopamine. It's the same rush that makes poker(slot) machines addictive - will the next spin hit the jackpot? This craving for unpredictability shows up in other places, too, scrolling social media for a funny video, a Netflix cliffhanger that finishes before you find out what happens, so you must watch the next episode, or on Tinder with the thrill of swiping till you find a new match. Our brains thrive on uncertainty, which fuels repeated engagement.

3. **Quick Repeatability**: The faster and easier it is to repeat a behaviour, the more it ingrains itself into our routines. With one quick click or swipe, you can play another round, watch another video, or get another match. Rapid repeatability reinforces the behaviour, cementing it into a habit.

These three components are why casinos and poker machines are so addictive. They offer continuous opportunity, unpredictable wins, and instant repeatability. Designed with the scarcity loop in mind, these environments exploit our brain's survival instincts, making us feel compelled to keep playing, even when it no longer serves us.

Understanding the scarcity loop empowers you to disrupt it. Humans are hardwired to respond to scarcity, but by redesigning our environment and habits, we can align our actions with our long-term goals and break free from the habits that undermine us.

To break free from this cycle, we can invert the Four Laws of Behaviour Change:

Stopping Unwanted Habits	
Inversion of the 1st law (Cue)	**Make it Invisible**
Inversion of the 2nd law (Craving)	**Make it Unattractive**
Inversion of the 3rd law (Response)	**Make it Difficult**
Inversion of the 4th law (Reward)	**Make it Unsatisfying**

Make it Invisible: Block the triggers that prompt the habit. You want to remove or minimise opportunities for the unwanted habit. This step alone can be overwhelming for some, but if it is out of sight, it is out of mind. It comes down to crafting the environmental conditions that help you make the change needed.

If you're prone to emotional snacking, keep tempting foods out of sight or out of your house altogether. If you can't stop picking up and mindlessly scrolling on your phone, delete the app from your phone. The fewer opportunities you have, the less often you'll engage.

Make it Unattractive: Impose an unattractive consequence for engaging with the unwanted behaviour, e.g., you eat a block of chocolate that is a 1-hour walk tomorrow. Try something more direct and put a picture of your fat self on the fridge so you remember why you are not going to eat those excess calories.

Reframe the behaviour so it loses its appeal. Think of the habit as an obstacle to your health and goals rather than a treat. Visualise the negative consequences rather than the fleeting reward.

Make it Difficult: To break the cycle of quick repeatability, add obstacles or friction to the behaviour. Adding a layer of difficulty disrupts the behaviour's automaticity.

If you are trying to reduce screen time, set a timer to lock the app after 15 minutes. Cancel your Netflix or Disney subscription. Don't bring home junk food or beer; instead, buy fruit and vegetables, salad and meat, so when you are hungry, your default is unprocessed, nutrient-dense food. Swap out the routine with one that gets you closer to your goal. Instead of snacking, call or text a friend, go for a walk or stretch. Find a calorie-negative behaviour to replace the calorie surplus behaviour.

Make it Unsatisfying: Create an accountability system that imposes a real cost for the behaviour. For instance, if you're trying to stop mindlessly scrolling on social media, commit to a friend or coach that each time you catch yourself scrolling, you'll give them $5. This consequence immediately makes the habit unsatisfying and interrupts the reward loop.

The other option that seems to be effective is to track the behaviour each time you do it. Keep a visible log on your phone, a notebook, or even a chart on the wall. Record when you do that behaviour and the time of day to help identify the trigger. This creates an immediate awareness of how frequently you engage in the habit, allowing you to see patterns and recognise the behaviour as a problem. Over time, this practice not only makes the habit less appealing but also helps build mindfulness around your actions, which is essential for change.

The key to establishing any new behaviour is to make it easy, obvious, and rewarding, but this takes planning and preparation. It will also take discipline and being cognizant of the triggers of unwanted habits. You must outsmart the behaviours that stop you from achieving your goal. Remember, willpower is limited, so creating an environment that supports you rather than inhibits you is vitally important.

The Power Of Your Environment

When trying to make behavioural changes, we can't rely on motivation or willpower because they are limited resources. Creating an environment that supports your efforts and applies the four laws of behaviour change is essential. If you can surround yourself with cues and rewards that reinforce your desired habits, you will have a much easier time getting the new habit to stick.

Imagine your bedroom, kitchen, lounge room, office, and gym are all designed to make good behaviours easier and bad behaviours harder. Making healthy choices becomes the default response to your environment. You don't need to motivate yourself constantly, it just becomes part of your routine. Take the time to create an environment filled with the right cues and people to ensure your road to success is not filled with potholes and setbacks.

If you want to explore habits in depth, I can't recommend Atomic Habits by James Clear strongly enough. It has helped me, and I have applied some of his ideas in this section.

"The environment is the invisible hand that shapes human behaviour" - James Clear.

Habit Hacking

Imagine your brain as a super-sophisticated computer with an amazing hard drive on which you can install any software programs you like that will shape your daily life. Your brain's structure and functions are the hardware, and your behaviours and language are the software.

Just like when you learn to use a new app on your phone, your brain learns habits through repetition and reinforcement. When you frequently choose to hit the snooze button instead of getting up on time, your brain starts running the snooze habit software. And just like a computer, the more you use a certain software, the more space it takes up in your brain's memory.

So, whether it's the positive habit of hitting the gym or cooking a healthy dinner or a negative habit of procrastinating with mindless scrolling, your brain's hardware gets wired with the software you feed it. It's like coding your operating system for life, one choice and one behaviour at a time.

Our brains are wired to seek evidence that confirms our beliefs, and our language can reinforce those beliefs, especially if they are limiting or negative. If you repeatedly tell yourself things like, "I'm not a morning person," "I can't do that," "I'm not that smart," or "I don't like vegetables," your brain will interpret those words as a script for its software, creating a reality where you are limited in those areas. To change the outcomes you get, you must rewrite the code.

Strategies to Help New Habits Take Hold

Implementation Intention

Imagine you're trying to implement a new self-improvement habit but keep getting to the end of the week, and it has yet to happen. You want to do it, but just can't find time to make it happen. Turns out, there's a smart way to make it happen reliably. Researchers discovered that if you pre-plan the what, when, and where you will include the new habit into your week, you are 2 to 3 times more likely to do it!

Fill in the gaps - **'I will [exercise/activity] on [day/time] at or in [place]'**

Creating an implementation plan lets you know exactly when, where, and how you will do said behaviour. Setting the intention doesn't leave things up to chance, meaning you don't have to find time or squeeze in a study, training or practice session; you have it set in your schedule.

Defining the what, when, and where removes the unknown factors and eliminates the anxiety that comes from knowing you have to do something but don't know where to start or how long it will take. Setting an implementation intention helps prepare you mentally (setting a clear intention) and physically (reduces anxiety) to remove the barriers to completing the desired behaviour.

Habit Stacking: Making Habits Work For You

Piggyback your desired new habit onto an existing daily habit to make adopting new behaviours easier and more efficient.

It is applying the 3rd Law of Behaviour Change - make it easy. Use existing behaviours as the trigger to start the new behaviour. For example, meditate right after brushing your teeth, make your tea or coffee in the morning, then go out into the sunshine or set your intentions for the day. You finish your training sessions and go to fill your water bottle (trigger) to leave, but instead of leaving, you go and do the cool-down stretches you always skip.

Unleash the transformative power of habit stacking by bundling up your habits like a pro.

Accountability Contracts: Don't Just Rely on Will-Power

You are striving to achieve great things and know the journey ahead will be long and challenging. What can you do to stay motivated and on track? Set up an Accountability contract.

Accountability contracts are formal agreements you make with yourself and/or others to follow through on a specific goal or habit. The primary purpose is to add a layer of social pressure and external motivation, which can significantly increase your likelihood of sticking to your commitments.

How to Use Accountability Contracts Effectively

Create a Clear and Specific Agreement: The contract should clearly outline the habit or goal, the timeline for achieving it, and the consequences if you don't follow through. The more specific the agreement, the more effective it becomes. It's crucial to define what failure looks like so you have a clear understanding of your target and everyone can recognise when commitments haven't been met. This clarity keeps you accountable and eliminates ambiguity, making it easier to stay on track and achieve your goals.

Involve an Accountability Partner: Share your contract with someone you trust - a friend, family member, or coach. This person will help hold you accountable by checking in on your progress and ensuring you adhere to the terms of your contract.

Set Up Consequences: Defining the stakes is an essential part of the contract. If you fail to meet your commitment, there should be a consequence. This could be anything from losing money to doing something you'd prefer not to. The idea is that the discomfort of the consequence outweighs the temptation to break the habit.

Make It Public: Sharing your accountability contract publicly, even with a small group, can increase your commitment. The more people know about your goals, the more pressure you feel to achieve them.

The 5-Minute Rule: Conquering Procrastination

What is the hardest part of a new behaviour? Getting started. The 5-minute rule tackles procrastination head-on. Commit to doing the task for just five minutes. That is it!

The idea is to make the task so easy that it's hard to say no. By committing to just five minutes, you lower the barrier to entry, making it less daunting to begin. Planning to stop after five minutes releases the worry and anxiety of getting through a whole session, but you are still adding the habit to your routine. The more familiar it becomes, the less inertia is required to engage in the new behaviours, and after a few sessions, you're in the groove and ready to keep going. Even if you stop after five minutes, you've still taken a meaningful step toward building that new habit and making it easier to return to next time.

Showing Up Counts: Build Self-Belief

Our actions either get us closer to or further away from our goals. Each time you choose to do something that aligns with your aspirations, you vote for the person you want to become. You reinforce that identity by going for your morning run, diving into a study session, attending a workshop, or preparing a healthy meal. The more votes you cast, the stronger the evidence becomes that you are an athlete, a dedicated scholar, or a healthy, fit individual. So, invest your energy in the behaviours that truly move the needle in the right direction, and you will be amazed at what you can accomplish and who you become.

4 Techniques For Upgrading Your Performance Software

Are you ready to unleash your potential? Buckle up because we're diving into the world of science-backed mental training and visualisation techniques that can take your performance and personal growth to a whole new level.

1. Mental Rehearsal: Pre-Event Visualisation & Imagery

At the start of the day, or before a game, training session, or performance, engage in mental rehearsal by closing your eyes and vividly visualising yourself succeeding. Picture each step, detail, and positive outcome as if you were already experiencing them. This anticipatory visualisation primes your mind for success, boosting confidence and performance when the moment arrives.

Visualisation creates a mental blueprint of success, which your brain then uses to guide your actions. For instance, athletes often use this technique to enhance their performance. Michael Phelps, the Olympic swimmer, famously visualised his races in detail before each competition, preparing his mind for every stroke and turn. Similarly, public speakers like Steve Jobs rehearsed their presentations extensively in their minds, ensuring smooth delivery and confidence on stage.

Imagine visualising yourself scoring the winning goal in a crucial game, executing perfect form during a training session, or delivering a flawless presentation at work. By mentally rehearsing these scenarios at the beginning of your day or right before the event, you condition your brain and body for the upcoming challenge. When the time comes, you're not overwhelmed because you've already "seen" the script play out in your mind. This mental preparation is a sneak peek into your future success, making the real experience more familiar and manageable.

Incorporating mental rehearsal and visualisation into your pre-event routine can transform your approach to challenges, turning uncertainty into a well-rehearsed performance and setting the stage for a successful outcome.

2. Rituals: Priming the Mind and Body

Rituals are more than just repetitive actions - they can be potent tools that ground you, enhance focus, and prime your mind for success. Whether preparing for a performance or navigating the high-pressure moments within an event, incorporating personal rituals can serve as psychological anchors, providing stability and control.

Rituals are intentional, specific behaviours or sequences of actions that can be used before any performance or during a game to prime your mind and body to execute the skill to the best of your ability. They are not random or arbitrary; they are deliberate practices aimed at enhancing focus, reducing anxiety, and preparing the body for the physical demands of competition.

For example, a tennis player might bounce the ball a certain number of times before serving, or a basketball player might go through a specific breathing routine before a free throw. These rituals help to create a sense of consistency and control, which can be especially important in high-pressure situations.

Moreover, rituals can serve as cues that signal the brain to enter a performance mindset. Whether placing water bottles in a specific order like Rafael Nadal or pulling up your socks before a shot at a goal, these actions become associated with success. They can help athletes get into the "zone" more consistently. They also provide a structured way to manage the unpredictable aspects of competition, offering a psychological anchor in high-stakes situations.

Superstitions, on the other hand, are behaviours that athletes believe bring them luck, but they do not directly influence their ability to perform. Common examples include wearing the same pair of socks for every game or not shaving during the playoffs. While these actions might provide a sense of comfort or confidence, they do not have a functional purpose related to the athlete's actual performance.

While superstitions can sometimes temporarily boost confidence, they can also become a hindrance if an athlete begins to rely on them too heavily. If a superstition is broken - the socks are unavailable - it can increase anxiety or decrease confidence, potentially undermining performance.

The key difference between rituals and superstitions lies in their intentionality and impact on performance. Rituals are purposeful actions to enhance performance through mental and physical preparation, while superstitions are comfort behaviours that have unknown outcomes on an athlete's performance.

Recognising this distinction is important for athletes who want to improve their game. While superstitions can boost confidence and reduce anxiety, they should not be relied upon as a primary performance strategy. Instead, athletes should focus on developing effective rituals that prime their minds and body for success, using these routines to establish control, focus, and readiness in high-pressure situations.

While both rituals and superstitions can affect an athlete's psychological state, rituals are the tools that directly influence performance by preparing the athlete to execute their skills at the highest level. Superstitions, while comforting, do not provide the same performance-enhancing benefits and should be viewed as secondary to the deliberate actions that make a difference on the field or court.

3. To Associate or Dissociate: A Mental Strategy for Improving Performance

When managing discomfort during high-performance situations like sports, exams, or public speaking, the mental strategies of association and dissociation come into play. This strategy determines whether to have a broad or narrow focus when dealing with stress, pain, or discomfort, often distinguishing between success and underperformance.

The association component is staying mentally engaged with the task and directly focusing on what your body or mind is experiencing. This method involves paying close attention to physical sensations, emotions, and thoughts, allowing for real-time adjustments and improvements.

For example, during a long-distance run, elite athletes often monitor their breathing, heart rate, muscle tension, and even environmental factors like wind resistance. They stay present with their bodies, using that data to control their pacing or adjust their technique to conserve energy. By staying connected to the experience, they manage discomfort by working with it rather than trying to block it out.

In everyday life, associating might involve focusing intently on your tonality and speed during a presentation. When discomfort arises (like nerves or a dry mouth), you don't panic or try to ignore it. Instead, you adjust - taking a sip of water or slowing down your speech to regain control.

Benefits of Association:

- Improved ability to adapt to challenges
- Enhanced body awareness and control
- Greater endurance under stressful conditions
- Ability to make real-time performance adjustments

Dissociation, conversely, involves diverting attention away from discomfort by mentally distancing yourself from the situation. This might mean distracting yourself with thoughts unrelated to the task at hand or focusing on external stimuli to avoid engaging with feelings of pain or stress.

For example, recreational runners often use dissociation, such as listening to music or daydreaming, to avoid thinking about fatigue or physical discomfort. This can be effective for shorter tasks, but it tends to reduce performance over time because it disconnects you from the signals your body is sending.

Benefits of Dissociation:

- Temporary relief from discomfort
- Increased ability to endure short-term stress
- A tool for distracting oneself from low-impact, routine tasks

When to Use Each Strategy:

Choosing between association and dissociation depends on the task at hand. Association is most effective during high-stakes situations that require attention to detail. It lets you stay connected to critical signals and make real-time adjustments to maintain optimal performance.

Dissociation, however, can be helpful when prolonged discomfort isn't a signal of danger or a need for adjustment, such as during a long hike, waiting in line, or engaging in repetitive menial tasks. It can also be useful when pushing through minor discomforts that don't require full attention.

4. Interpreting Feelings: Messengers or Dictators?

How you handle your feelings can make or break your performance in a performance arena. Understanding the role of feelings is crucial for performance. Feelings can be powerful influencers in your performance, but the key lies in whether you allow them to serve as messengers that inform your actions or dictators that control them. The difference between these two approaches can significantly impact your ability to perform under pressure.

Messengers: Inform, Don't Control

If you start feeling fatigued during a marathon, this doesn't mean you should give up. Instead, interpret the fatigue as a cue to adjust your pace and take in some fluids to ensure you finish. Treating your feelings as messengers gives you valuable insights into how your body responds and can make adjustments to optimise your performance.

When you tune into your emotions, you better understand how they correlate with your performance. This self-awareness helps you identify patterns, like how a bit of nervous energy can improve your focus or reaction time or how frustration and anger are signs that you need to change your approach.

Feelings as Dictators: When Emotions Take Over

On the flip side, when feelings become dictators, they control your actions, often leading to impulsive or destructive behaviour:

Loss of Focus: Frustration during a match might cause you to lash out, leading to mistakes that could have been avoided.

Clouded Judgment: Strong emotions can distort perception, leading to poor decisions, such as playing too conservatively out of fear or taking unnecessary risks out of anger.

Limited Growth: Letting feelings dictate your actions can cause you to avoid challenges, limiting your potential to grow and improve.

In the end, feelings can either be powerful tools that guide your actions or obstacles that hinder your progress. By treating feelings as messengers rather than dictators, you take control of your emotional responses, allowing you to make decisions that align with your goals. This mindset shift enables you to stay focused, make informed decisions, and push through challenges, ultimately leading to improved performance in all areas of life.

Tools To Help Get Things Done

The 5-Second Rule: 5, 4, 3, 2, 1- GO

The 5-Second Rule is a powerful and straightforward tool for taking immediate action, especially when procrastination or hesitation threatens to derail your progress. The technique involves counting down from five to one and then launching into whatever action you need to take. This simple act interrupts the habit of overthinking and forces you to commit to action within five seconds.

Why It Works: The countdown interrupts your brain's natural tendency to talk you out of doing something uncomfortable or challenging. By counting backward, you engage the prefrontal cortex, the part of the brain responsible for decision-making and logical thinking. This activation helps to override the limbic system, which is responsible for emotions and behaviours and can often lead to procrastination or inaction.

Boost Productivity: Whether you're trying to get into a cold bath, start a workout, stop scrolling or tackle a tough task at work, the 5-Second Rule can help you overcome resistance and take immediate action.

Combat Distractions: It effectively breaks the cycle of mindless scrolling or unproductive behaviours. For instance, if you find yourself endlessly scrolling through social media, you can use the rule to stop: say to yourself, "I'm going to close the app in 5, 4, 3, 2, 1", and then follow through. This breaks the spell of digital distractions and helps you refocus on tasks that align with your goals.

Build Momentum: Once you've started, the hardest part is over. The initial action often leads to further progress, creating momentum that propels you forward. Even if the action is small, like putting down your phone or opening a book to study, it's a crucial first step that moves you closer to your goals.

The beauty of the 5-Second Rule is in its simplicity and accessibility. You don't need special tools or extensive training to use it, just the willingness to count down and take action. It's a versatile technique that can be applied in countless situations to help you start doing the habits that will move you toward your goals.

Pomodoro Technique

The Pomodoro Technique is a time management strategy that breaks work into focused intervals, typically 25 minutes long, known as "Pomodoros." After each Pomodoro, you take a short break, e.g. 5 minutes to recharge. After completing four Pomodoros, you reward yourself with a longer break. This technique leverages the brain's natural ability to concentrate for short bursts, boosting productivity while preventing burnout and ensuring steady, consistent progress.

Task Prioritisation and To-Do Lists

Being busy doesn't always mean being productive. To truly move the needle toward your goals, it's essential to prioritise tasks that matter rather than getting caught up in activities that fill your time. Effective time management begins with task prioritisation, which ensures that your efforts are aligned with your most important objectives.

One powerful tool for this is the Time Management Matrix, which helps you categorise tasks by urgency and importance. By distinguishing between what's truly critical and what needs to be done but is not urgent, you can create a more focused and efficient workflow.

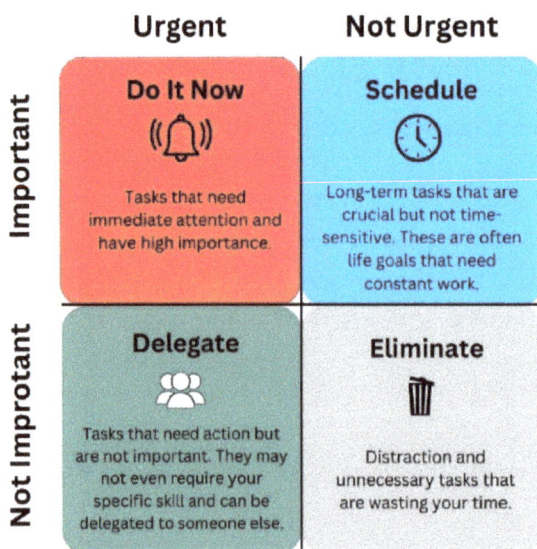

	Urgent	Not Urgent
Important	**Do It Now** Tasks that need immediate attention and have high importance.	**Schedule** Long-term tasks that are crucial but not time-sensitive. These are often life goals that need constant work.
Not Important	**Delegate** Tasks that need action but are not important. They may not even require your specific skill and can be delegated to someone else.	**Eliminate** Distraction and unnecessary tasks that are wasting your time.

How to Use: Draw a 4-quadrant box and label Urgent/Not Urgent and Important/Not Important.

1. Urgent and Important: These tasks require immediate attention and have significant consequences if not completed. They should be your top priority.

2. Important but Not Urgent: These tasks are crucial for long-term goals but don't need immediate action - schedule time for these to ensure steady progress.

3. Urgent but Not Important: Tasks that demand attention now but don't significantly contribute to your goals. Delegate these or set limits on how much time you spend on them.

4. Neither Urgent nor Important: Tasks that don't advance your goals and are often distractions. Minimise or eliminate these from your day.

Once you have prioritised the tasks that are important to your goals, create a to-do list for the day or week. This will help you know where to focus your efforts and avoid wasting time on aimless activities.

Time Blocking and Scheduling

Now that you know what you need to work on, block out time to dedicate to the specific tasks or activities. Create a structured schedule that includes work tasks, breaks, exercise, personal time, etc. By allocating time for each activity, you reduce ambiguity and ensure that essential tasks are addressed. Stick to your schedule as closely as possible to minimise unproductive gaps.

Digital Detox and Distraction Management

In today's digital age, distractions from smartphones, social media, and online content are major productivity inhibitors. Implement a digital detox by setting specific times for checking emails and notifications. Consider using apps or browser extensions that block distracting websites during work periods. Set a timer on your social apps on your phone so you stop mindless scrolling after 15 minutes. Disconnecting from these distractions enhances focus and productivity.

Remember, the effectiveness of these tools and habits can vary from person to person. Experimenting and tailoring these strategies to your unique working style and preferences is essential. Overcoming procrastination and enhancing productivity often require consistent practice and adjustments to find what works best for you.

You are armed with the toolkit to boost your brainpower and productivity. So, embrace these techniques and watch your life go from good to great.

Part 3 - Three Layers of Behaviour Change - Start From The Inside Out

Imagine you're a sculptor, chiselling away at a massive block of marble. Your goal? To transform that block into a magnificent statue. The process is similar to changing your behaviours. It involves peeling back layers and refining your work until your masterpiece emerges.

Establishing long-lasting and effective behaviour change is not easy, but knowing where to hit with the chisel creates the masterpiece. To create the best version of yourself, let's dive into the three layers of behaviour change.

Three Layers Of Behaviour Change

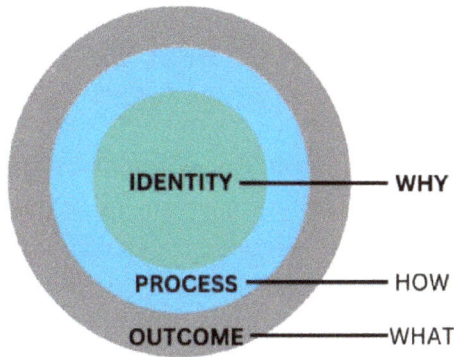

The Outer Layer: Defining Outcomes

The first layer is like the rough outline of your sculpture. This layer is concerned with changing your results, much like your raw vision of what the statue might look like. Losing weight, graduating from university, winning a championship - these are the Outcome goals you set for yourself. Nothing really changes here, but it outlines the destination.

The Middle Layer: Changing Your Systems and Environment

You know what you want, but how do you get there? The second layer is changing your habits, systems, and environment. For example, implementing a new gym routine, decluttering your desk for a better workflow, or developing a meditation practice. This layer is all about the habits and systems you build and refine over time.

The Core Layer: Creating A New Identity

You won't be able to improve your health, performance, sleep, etc., if you drag your old habits and behaviours behind you like an anchor. Changing your behaviours and, ultimately, your identity will require you to look inside and uncover who you want to be and how you see yourself in the world. These identity-based habits are the final layer you etch into your sculpture, the deepest layer where you uncover the identity of who you want to become. It's about changing your beliefs, self-image, and actions to become the person you know you can be.

The Power Of Identity Change: Becoming Who You Aspire to Be

Aligning your identity with the person you aspire to become is the foundation of true and lasting behaviour change. It's not just about altering your habits or tweaking your mindset but fundamentally transforming how you see yourself. When your identity aligns with your aspirations, every decision you make supports your journey toward becoming that person.

If you are unsure what behaviours to embrace, find someone already with the results, physique, or position you want to be in and watch how they behave and make decisions. This will help you align your behaviours with the person you strive to become. For instance, if you aim to be a professional athlete, study how they manage their time, approach their training, and handle setbacks. Emulating their actions can guide your own behaviour, reinforcing the decisions and behaviours you need to adopt.

Imagine this: You're out with friends, deciding what to eat. If you see yourself as fit and healthy, your choice naturally aligns with that identity. You opt for steak and vegetables instead of burgers and chips because that's what a healthy person would do. This isn't about willpower or self-denial; it's about embodying the identity of someone who prioritises their health and wants to nourish their body.

For example, you're an aspiring triathlete invited to a friend's place for a few beers after work. But you identify as a professional athlete in training. What would a professional do? You hit the gym instead because that choice aligns with the identity you've embraced. No matter how big or small, each decision is a vote for the person you're striving to become.

Similarly, if you identify as someone with a specific skill set - playing a musical instrument, mastering a sport, or excelling in a particular field, you naturally prioritise time to practice and hone that skill. This becomes a part of your identity. For example, if you see yourself as a dedicated guitarist, you find time every day to practice, no matter how busy your schedule is. Practising isn't just an activity; it reflects who you are. You train your skills because it's integral to your identity, not just something you do occasionally.

This shift in identity creates a powerful framework for decision-making. When you see yourself as someone with more muscles than body fat, you naturally engage in behaviours to maintain this identity. Your identity becomes the compass guiding your choices, ensuring that your actions align with your goals.

But it doesn't stop there. This identity shift influences all three layers of behaviour change. When your identity is aligned with your aspirations, you start to shape an environment that supports those goals. You surround yourself with influences that uplift and reinforce your new identity, whether it's the people you spend time with or the routines you establish.

When all three layers are in harmony, you're not leaving things up to chance. You are in control of your destiny. You become the embodiment of your aspirations, and this holistic approach propels you toward becoming the best version of yourself, whether as an athlete, performer or simply a healthier individual.

Remember, your journey to success is ongoing, and setbacks are inevitable. But when your identity is aligned with your goals, you have the resilience and mindset to overcome challenges. You're not just hoping to become the person you want to be - you're already that person, and every action you take reinforces that. This is the power of identity change: it allows you to embody the transformation you seek, making your goals achievable and inevitable.

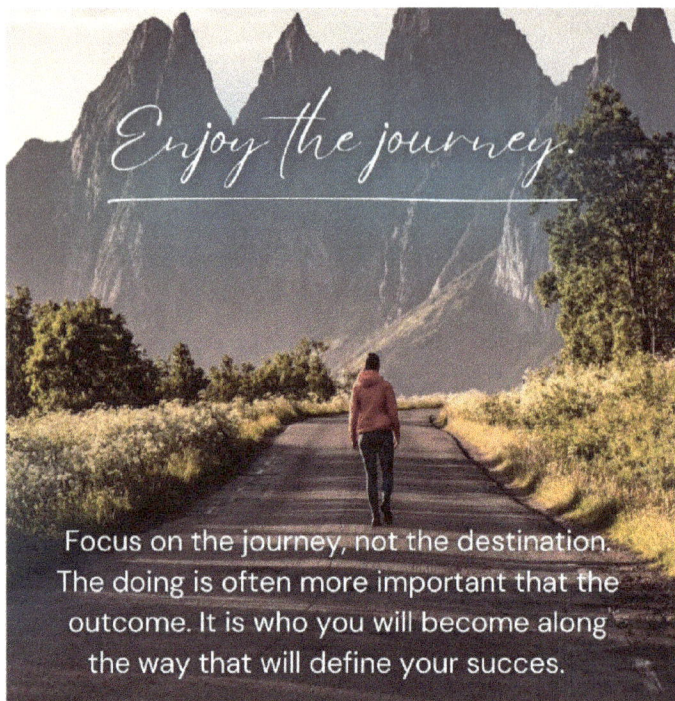

Focus on the journey, not the destination. The doing is often more important that the outcome. It is who you will become along the way that will define your succes.

Mastering New Skills In Just 20 Hours

Now, imagine acquiring any skill you desire in just 20 hours. Does that sound too good to be true? Well, the science behind deliberate practice proves that it is possible. The secret lies in breaking down the skill into its fundamental building blocks and mastering each one.

It's like learning to play a musical instrument. You don't start by trying to master a complex piece of music. You start by learning the basics - the notes, the scales, the chords. Once you've mastered these smaller skills, you can combine them to play the music. This is the power of deliberate practice.

I'm sure you have heard the saying, 'Practice Makes Perfect,' but the reality is, **'Perfect Practice Makes Perfect'**. This is why deliberate, focused practice is required to master skills.

This is the power of being clear about what you want to achieve, allocating time each week, and doing deliberate, focused practice. Once you master one skill, move on to the next, and you will be able to build a comprehensive set of skills and, over time, achieve great things.

How Long Does It Take To Form A New Habit?

The timeline for forming a new habit can vary widely among individuals, and research suggests that there is no one-size-fits-all answer. The idea that it takes 21 days to form a habit originated from a misinterpretation of a study by Dr Maxwell Maltz in the 1960s. More recent research provides a more nuanced understanding of habit formation. Studies on habit formation have shown a range of time frames, and no consensus exists on a specific duration.

Various factors, including the complexity of the behaviour, individual differences, motivation, and repetition frequency, influence the time it takes to form a habit. Here are some key points from the research:

Variability in Duration: A 2009 study found that, on average, it took participants about 66 days to establish a new habit. However, the time frame varied widely, with some participants taking as little as 18 days and others as long as 254 days.

Behaviour Complexity Matters: The complexity of the behaviour influences the time it takes to form a habit. Simple behaviours might become habits more quickly than complex ones.

Consistency is Key: Repetition and consistency are crucial for habit formation. The more consistently a behaviour is repeated, the more likely it becomes a habit.

Individual Differences: Individual factors, such as personality, motivation, and the perceived difficulty of the behaviour, affect how quickly a habit is formed.

Environmental Design: The easier and faster you can repeat the behaviour, the more likely you are to repeat it - for both good and bad.

Crafting the environment to facilitate the desired behaviour will increase habit formation.

It's important to recognise that habit formation is not a one-size-fits-all process. While the idea of a 21-day rule has become popular, research shows that forming a new habit is a deeply personal journey shaped by various factors unique to each individual. The key to successfully establishing and mastering new habits and skills is not the timeline but the consistency and repetition of the habits and specific skills.

Closing: The Journey To Success

Success is something we all desire, yet it's often misunderstood. Success isn't something you chase - it's something you attract by the person you become. The more you chase it, the more elusive it feels. But when you shift your focus to developing yourself, success naturally finds its way to you.

It starts with a simple question: What kind of person are you becoming? Success is attracted to qualities like discipline, integrity, perseverance, and generosity. It's drawn to people who are intentional about their lives, who set clear goals, and who take consistent action toward those goals.

The truth is, success requires a price: time, effort, discipline, and sacrifice. But it's not about waiting for circumstances to change, it's about changing yourself. As Jim Rohn once said, *"If you want things to change, you have to change. If you want things to get better, you have to get better."*

This journey starts with your habits. Your daily habits shape your future. Success isn't built on occasional effort, it's the result of consistent, intentional action. It's about showing up every day, even when it's hard, and committing to the process of growth.

Equally important is your mindset. Your mindset is the foundation upon which success is built. If your thoughts are filled with doubt, fear, and limiting beliefs, success will be out of reach. But when you believe in your ability to grow, to improve, and to achieve, you lay the groundwork for transformation. Surround yourself with positive influences, seek inspiration, and feed your mind with empowering thoughts.

Finally, remember the power of your relationships. Surround yourself with people who inspire you, who challenge you to be better, and who align with your vision. As the saying goes, *"Show me your friends, and I'll show you your future."*

Success isn't about luck or shortcuts, it's about who you become through discipline, consistency, and belief. As you close this book, take the first step: define your goals, align your habits, and commit to becoming the best version of yourself. Because when you change, everything changes.

The journey to success is yours to take. Now go make it happen!

The Final Challenge - Habits And Behaviours For Success

In this final challenge, I have raised the bar to ensure you implement the lessons in this book and begin making real progress toward your goals. This time, there are eight practical challenges to help you solidify new habits and behaviours and set yourself up for long-term success.

Level 1: Master Goal Setting for Success

Follow the 4-step process to set clear and actionable goals:

1. **Establish Long-Term Outcome Goals:** Define what you want to achieve in the next 1–5 years.

2. **Identify Learning Goals:** Pinpoint the skills or knowledge you need to acquire to achieve those long-term goals.

3. **Set Performance Goals:** Break your outcome goals into medium-term, measurable milestones (e.g., quarterly or monthly).

4. **Outline Process Goals:** Identify the short-term, daily or weekly habits that will move you toward your performance goals.

5. **Create a Goal Tracker:** Use a journal, app, or spreadsheet to track your progress and review it weekly to stay on course.

Level 2: Introduce a Keystone Habit

Identify **one powerful habit** that will create a ripple effect on other areas of your life (e.g., daily exercise, meal prep, or journaling).

Implement the habit using the **Four Laws of Habit Formation**:

1. **Make it Obvious:** Keep cues visible and consistent (e.g., leave workout clothes out at night).

2. **Make it Attractive:** Pair the habit with something enjoyable (e.g., listen to your favourite podcast while walking).

3. **Make it Easy:** Start small and build up (e.g., a 5-minute habit to begin).

4. **Make it Satisfying:** Reward yourself for completing the habit (e.g., check it off your tracker).

Level 3: Take Immediate Action

Pick **one action** you can take right now to move closer to your goals. Whether it's signing up for a course, clearing your pantry of junk food, or creating your goal tracker, **do it today.** Small, immediate action builds momentum.

Level 4: Weekly Review and Reflection

At the end of each week, take 15 minutes to:

- **Review your progress:** What habits worked? What didn't?

- **Adjust as needed:** Identify obstacles and tweak your environment or process goals.

- **Celebrate small wins:** Acknowledge even the smallest successes to build momentum.

Level 5: Create a Winning Environment

Your environment either supports or sabotages your habits. Make intentional changes:

- **At Home:** Stock healthy foods, designate clutter-free zones for work, and eliminate distractions.

- **At Work:** Create a workspace free from temptations, turn off unnecessary notifications, and surround yourself with tools that enhance productivity.

- **Social Environment:** Spend time with people who align with your goals and inspire you to grow. Reduce exposure to negative influences.

Level 6: Create a Vision Board

- Use tools like Canva (free and easy) or physical materials (magazines, markers, etc.) to create a **visual representation of your goals.** Include images, quotes, and milestones that represent the life you want to achieve.

- Place the vision board somewhere you'll see it daily to keep your goals top of mind.

Level 7: Habit Stacking for Excellence

Stack your new habit onto an existing one to ensure it sticks. For example:

- After brushing your teeth (existing habit), meditate for 5 minutes (new habit).

- After brewing your morning tea or coffee (existing habit), set your intentions for the day (new habit).

Level 8: Accountability and Feedback

- Share your goals with someone who can hold you accountable (a friend, mentor, or coach).

- Send me an email at **josh@healthwealthgroup.com.au** or leave a review on Amazon. Share what you found valuable, what changes you've made, and the successes you've achieved. Your feedback not only inspires others but keeps you accountable.

Take action, start today, and commit to your journey of growth and success.

Congratulations On Completing The Book!

Take a moment to reflect upon all you have learned and how you can apply it. I hope you can use the tools and strategies found in this book to unlock the doors to your dreams. Believe with all your heart that your goals and ambitions are attainable.

Picture this: You are at a crossroads, deciding the direction your life will take. But now, you're equipped with the tools and knowledge to navigate your way to success. Do you stay on the highway that everyone travels - a road leading to a life of quiet desperation? Or do you choose the unknown route, embarking on an adventure to reach your true potential?

My final words to you are this: Your outcomes are defined by your inputs. The results you want are shaped by your choices, the sacrifices you're willing to endure, and the effort you put in each day. Great achievements require great effort, but with consistency, resilience, and determination, they are within your reach. Take charge and be the lead character in your story - don't be a spectator.

I wish you all the best on your journey to greatness and look forward to hearing about your success.

Be the best you can be,

Josh Euler

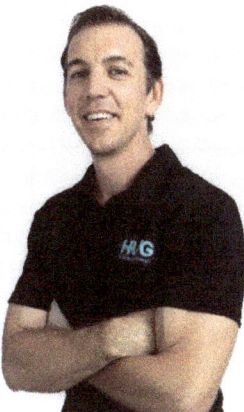

Attributions

Concepts and portions of this text have been taken from the following books. I recommend reading or listening to these books to help you on your journey to greatness.

Trevor Moward - It Takes What It Takes

Viktor E Frankl - Man's Search For Meaning

Robert Sapolsky - Why Zebras Don't Get Ulcers

Dr Melissa Davis - Evidence Based Habit Building

James Clear - Atomic Habits

Charles Duhigg - The Power of Habit

Stephen R Covey - The 7 Habits of Highly Successful People

Amishi Jha - Peak Mind

Rich Diviney - The Attributes

John C Maxwell - Change Your World

Dr Matthew Walker - Why We Sleep: Unlocking the Power of Sleep and Dreams

Michael Pollan - In Defense of Foods

Steven Kotler - The Art of Impossible

George Mumford - The Mindful Athlete

Dr Joe Dispenza - Becoming Supernatural

Shawn Stevenson - Eat Smarter

Tim S. Grover - Relentless

Steve Magness - Do Hard Things

Simon Quellen Field - Gut Reactions: The Science Of Weight Gain and Loss

Michael Easter - The Scarcity Brain

References

Minges KE, Redeker NS. Delayed school start times and adolescent sleep: A systematic review of the experimental evidence. Sleep. 2020;43(12):zsaa140. doi: 10.1093/sleep/zsaa140.

Sprajcer M, Dawson D, Kosmadopoulos A, Sach EJ, Crowther ME, Sargent C, Roach GD. (2023). How Tired is Too Tired to Drive? A Systematic Review Assessing the Use of Prior Sleep Duration to Detect Driving Impairment. Nature and Science of Sleep, 15, 175–206. https://doi.org/10.2147/NSS.S392441

Van den Berg L, Blanken TF, Van der Ende J, et al. The longitudinal association between sleep quality and symptoms of anxiety and depression in adolescence. Journal of Adolescent Health. 2021;68(4):774-780. doi: 10.1016/j.jadohealth.2020.12.023.

Suh S, Paik I, Shin C. Inadequate sleep and adolescent obesity: The Korean National Health and Nutrition Examination Survey 2013-2014. Pediatrics. 2020;145(2):e20191600. doi: 10.1542/peds.2019-1600.

Harvard Health Publishing. (2019). Sleep and mental health. https://www.health.harvard.edu/newsletter_article/sleep-and-mental-health

Baglioni, C., Nanovska, S., Regen, W., Spiegelhalder, K., Feige, B., Nissen, C., & Riemann, D. (2016). Sleep and mental disorders: A meta-analysis of polysomnographic research. Psychological Bulletin, 142(9), 969-990.

Trexler ET, et al. International society of sports nutrition position stand: Beta-Alanine. J Int Soc Sports Nutr. 2015;12:30.

International society of sports nutrition position stand: caffeine and performance. J Int Soc Sports Nutr. 2010;7:5. doi: 10.1186/1550-2783-7-5.

Schwedhelm, E., Maas, R., Freese, R., Jung, D., Lukacs, Z., Jambrecina, A., & Böger, R. H. (2008). Pharmacokinetic and pharmacodynamic properties of oral L-citrulline and L-arginine: impact on nitric oxide metabolism. British Journal of Clinical Pharmacology, 65(1), 51–59.

Phillips SM, et al. The role of milk- and soy-based protein in support of muscle protein synthesis and muscle protein accretion in young and elderly persons. J Am Coll Nutr. 2009;28(4):343-354.

Tartibian B, et al. Omega-3 fatty acids supplementation attenuates inflammatory markers after eccentric exercise in untrained men. Clin J Sport Med. 2011;21(2):131-137.

Coker, N. (2020, November 13). What's Better: L-Citrulline or Citrulline Malate? Retrieved from https://www.bodybuilding.com/content/l-citrulline-or-citrulline-malate-n-o-content.html

Goldstein ER, et al. International society of sports nutrition position stand: caffeine and performance. J Int Soc Sports Nutr. 2010;7:5.

Morton, R.W., Murphy, K.T., McKellar, S.R., Schoenfeld, B.J., Henselmans, M., Helms, E., Aragon, A.A., Devries, M.C., Banfield, L., Krieger, J.W. and Phillips, S.M., 2018. A systematic review, meta-analysis and meta-regression of the effect of protein supplementation on resistance training-induced gains in muscle mass and strength in healthy adults. Journal of the International Society of Sports Nutrition, 15(1), p.15. Available at: https://jissn.biomedcentral.com/articles/10.1186/s12970-018-0215-1

Grandjean AC, et al. Dehydration and cognitive performance. J Am Coll Nutr. 2007;26(5 Suppl):549S-554S.

Adan A. Cognitive performance and dehydration. J Am Coll Nutr. 2012;31(2):71-78.

Cheuvront SN, et al. Hydration assessment of athletes. Sports Med. 2010;40(1):23-41.

Sawka MN, et al. American College of Sports Medicine position stand. Exercise and fluid replacement. Med Sci Sports Exerc. 2007;39(2):377-390.

Institute of Medicine. Dietary Reference Intakes for Water, Potassium, Sodium, Chloride, and Sulfate. Washington, DC: The National Academies Press; 2005.

Grandner, M. A., Jackson, N., Gerstner, J. R., & Knutson, K. L. (2014). Sleep symptoms associated with intake of specific dietary nutrients. Journal of Sleep Research, 23(1), 22-34.

Sexton, C. E., Storsve, A. B., & Walhovd, K. B. (2017). Johanneberg Science Park, Gothenburg, Sweden. Sleep, 40(suppl_1), A376-A376.

Besedovsky, L., Lange, T., & Born, J. (2012). Sleep and immune function. Pflügers Archiv-European Journal of Physiology, 463(1), 121-137.

Cappuccio, F. P., D'Elia, L., Strazzullo, P., & Miller, M. A. (2010). Sleep duration and all-cause mortality: a systematic review and meta-analysis of prospective studies. Sleep, 33(5), 585-592.

Taheri, S., Lin, L., Austin, D., Young, T., & Mignot, E. (2004). Short sleep duration is associated with reduced leptin, elevated ghrelin, and increased body mass index. PLoS medicine, 1(3), e62.

Mah, C. D., Mah, K. E., Kezirian, E. J., & Dement, W. C. (2011). The effects of sleep extension on the athletic performance of collegiate basketball players. Sleep, 34(7), 943-950.

Diekelmann, S., & Born, J. (2010). The memory function of sleep. Nature Reviews Neuroscience, 11(2), 114-126.

Haack, M., & Mullington, J. M. (2005). Sustained sleep restriction reduces emotional and physical well-being. Pain, 119(1-3), 56-64.

Dupuy, O., Douzi, W., Theurot, D., Bosquet, L., & Dugué, B. (2018). An Evidence-Based Approach for Choosing Post-exercise Recovery Techniques to Reduce Markers of Muscle Damage, Soreness, Fatigue, and Inflammation: A Systematic Review With Meta-Analysis. Frontiers in Physiology, 9, 403. doi: 10.3389/fphys.2018.00403. PMID: 29755363. PMCID: PMC5932411. https://www.ncbi.nlm.nih.gov/pmc/articles/PMC5932411/

Human Kinetics. (2021, July 15). What are the best recovery strategies for athletes? https://humankinetics.me/2021/07/15/what-are-the-best-recovery-strategies-for-athletes/

Kreider RB, et al. ISSN exercise & sports nutrition review update: research & recommendations. J Int Soc Sports Nutrition. 2010;7:7.

Cunha, L. A., Costa, J. A., Marques, E. A., Brito, J., Lastella, M., & Figueiredo, P. (2023). The Impact of Sleep Interventions on Athletic Performance: A Systematic Review. Sports Medicine - Open, 9(1), 1-18. https://doi.org/10.1186/s40798 -023-00599-z

Fry, A., & Rehman, A. (2022) Physical Activity and Sleep: Athletic Performance and Recovery. Retrieved from https://www.sleepfoundation.org/physical. -activity/athletic-performance-and-sleep#references-79290

Healthline, Kerri Ann, J, (2023). 11 Brain Foods: Boost Memory, Focus, and Mental Clarity. Retrieved from https://www.healthline.com/nutrition/11-brain-foods

www.ingramcontent.com/pod-product-compliance
Lightning Source LLC
Chambersburg PA
CBHW052011030426
42334CB00029BA/3172